POCKET COMPANION FOR

Physical Examination & Health Assessment

3rd *Canadian Edition*

Carolyn Jarvis, PhD, APN, CNP

Professor of Nursing
School of Nursing
Illinois Wesleyan University
Bloomington, Illinois;

and

Family Nurse Practitioner
Bloomington, Illinois

Canadian Editors

Annette J. Browne, RN, PhD
Professor & Distinguished
University Scholar
School of Nursing
University of British
Columbia
Vancouver, British Columbia

June MacDonald-Jenkins, RN, BScN, MSc
Dean, School of Health, Human
& Justice Studies
Loyalist College
Belleville, Ontario

Marian Luctkar-Flude, RN, PhD
Assistant Professor
School of Nursing
Queen's University
Kingston, Ontario

Original Illustrations by
Pat Thomas, CMI, FAMI
East Troy, Wisconsin

Assessment Photographs by
Kevin Strandberg
Professor of Art
Illinois Wesleyan University
Bloomington, Illinois

ELSEVIER

ELSEVIER

POCKET COMPANION FOR PHYSICAL EXAMINATION
& HEALTH ASSESSMENT, THIRD CANADIAN EDITION   ISBN: 978-1-771-72149-3

Notices

Practitioners and researchers must always rely on their own experience and knowledge in evaluating and using any information, methods, compounds or experiments
described herein. Because of rapid advances in the medical sciences, in particular,
independent verification of diagnoses and drug dosages should be made. To the
fullest extent of the law, no responsibility is assumed by Elsevier, authors, editors
or contributors for any injury and/or damage to persons or property as a matter
of products liability, negligence or otherwise, or from any use or operation of any
methods, products, instructions, or ideas contained in the material herein.

Library of Congress Control Number: 2018959643

VP Education Content: Kevonne Holloway
Content Strategist, Canada Acquisitions: Roberta A. Spinosa-Millman
Senior Content Development Specialist: Heather Bays
Publishing Services Manager: Deepthi Unni
Project Manager: Srividhya Vidhyashankar

Working together
to grow libraries in
developing countries

www.elsevier.com • www.bookaid.org

Last digit is the print number: 9 8 7 6 5 4 3 2 1

Preface

The third edition of *Pocket Companion for Physical Examination and Health Assessment* is designed for two groups—those who need a practical clinical reference and those acquiring beginning assessment skills.

First, the *Pocket Companion* is intended as an adjunct to Jarvis' *Physical Examination and Health Assessment*, 3rd Canadian edition. The *Pocket Companion* is a memory prompt for those who have studied physical assessment and wish to have a reminder when in the clinic. The *Pocket Companion* has all the essentials: health history points, exam steps for each body system, normal versus abnormal findings, heart sounds, lung sounds, and neurologic checks. *The Pocket Companion* is useful when you forget a step in the exam sequence, when you wish to be sure your assessment is complete, when you need to review the findings that are normal versus abnormal, or when you are faced with an unfamiliar technique or a new clinical area. Its portable size and binding make it perfect for a lab coat pocket or community health bag.

Second, the *Pocket Companion*, 3rd Canadian edition, is an independent primer of basic assessment skills. It is well suited to programs offering a beginning assessment course covering well people of all ages. The *Pocket Companion* has the complete steps to perform a health history and physical examination on a well person. It includes pertinent developmental content for pediatric, pregnant, and aging adult patients. Although the description

of each exam step is stated concisely, there is enough information given to study and learn exam techniques. However, since there is no room in the *Pocket Companion* for theories, principles, or detailed explanations, students using the *Pocket Companion* as a beginning text must have a thorough didactic presentation of assessment methods as well as tutored practice.

The *Pocket Companion*, 3rd Canadian edition, is revised and updated to match the revision of the parent text, *Physical Examination and Health Assessment*, 3rd Canadian edition, including many new examination photos, abnormal findings photos, and full-color art.

A new section on the **Electronic Health Record** has been integrated into Chapter 21, Bedside Assessment and Electronic Health Recording. This section outlines charting, and narrative recording provides examples of how to document assessment findings.

For those times when readers need detailed coverage of a particular technique or finding, it is easily found through numerous cross-references to pages in *Physical Examination and Health Assessment*, 3rd Canadian edition.

As you thumb through the *Pocket Companion*, note these features:
- Health history and exam steps are concise yet complete.
- Method of examination is clear, orderly, and easy to follow.
- Abnormal findings are described briefly in a column adjacent to the normal range of findings.

- Sample charting is now included in all applicable chapters, illustrating the documentation of findings.
- Tables are presented at the end of chapters to fully illustrate important information.
- Selected Cultural Competencies information highlights this important aspect of a health assessment.
- Developmental Competencies content includes age-specific information for pediatric, pregnant, and aging adult groups.
- Summary checklists for each chapter form a cue card of exam steps to remember.
- Integration of the complete physical examination is presented in Chapter 20.
- Selected artwork from *Physical Examination and Health Assessment*, 3rd Canadian edition, illustrates the pertinent anatomy.

ACKNOWLEDGMENTS

I am grateful to those on the team at Elsevier who worked on the *Pocket Companion*. My thanks extend to Lee Henderson, Content Strategist; Laurie Gower, Content Manager; Heather Bays, Senior Development Specialist; and Brandi Flagg, Senior Production Manager, for their patient and attentive monitoring of every step in the production of the *Pocket Companion*.

Carolyn Jarvis

The Canadian editors are grateful for the support of the Elsevier staff, especially the Content Strategist, Roberta Spinosa-Millman; the Developmental Editor, Heather Bays; and freelance editor, Tammy Scherer. We would also like to thank all of the Canadian contributors who made the third Canadian edition of the *Physical Examination & Health Assessment* textbook and the third edition of this *Pocket Companion* possible.

Annette J. Browne
June MacDonald-Jenkins
Marian Luctkar-Flude

Contents

Contents

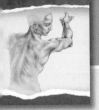
The Interview and the Complete Health History

Both the interview and the health history entail the collection of **subjective data**: what the patient says about herself, himself, or themselves. The interview is the optimal way to learn about the patient's perceptions of, understandings of, and reactions to their health state, which includes physical, mental, spiritual, and emotional health. The goal of this meeting is to record a complete health history.

The health history helps you begin to identify the patient's health strengths and problems and contextual influences, and it functions as a bridge to the next step in data collection: the physical examination. The history is combined with the **objective data** from the physical examination and with laboratory results to form the database used to make a judgement or diagnosis about an individual's health status.

ATTENDING TO THE PHYSICAL SETTING

Ensuring Privacy

Aim for geographical privacy; ideally, a private space. If geographical privacy is not available, "psychological privacy" by curtained partitions may suffice as long as the patient feels sure no one can overhear the conversation or interrupt.

Refusing Interruptions

You need to concentrate and to establish rapport.

Physical Environment

- Make the distance between you and the patient about 1.5 m (twice arm's length).
- Arrange equal-status seating. Both you and the patient should be comfortably seated, at eye level with each other. Avoid facing a patient across a desk or table because that feels like a barrier.
- Avoid standing over the patient.

There are three phases to each interview: an introduction, a working phase, and a termination (or closing).

INTRODUCING THE INTERVIEW

Address the patient, using the patient's surname, and shake hands if that seems appropriate to the context and the patient, and if it feels comfortable. Introduce yourself and state your role in the agency (if you are a student, say so). If you are gathering a complete history, give the reason for this interview (e.g., "Mr. Yuan, I would like to ask you some questions about your health and your usual daily activities so that we can plan your care here in the hospital.").

THE WORKING PHASE

The working phase is the data-gathering phase. Verbal skills for this phase include your questions to the patient and your responses to what the patient has said. Two types of questions exist: open-ended and closed. Each

1

type has a different place and function in the interview.

Open-Ended Questions

The **open-ended question** asks for narrative information. The topic to be discussed is stated, but only in general terms. Use it to begin the interview, to introduce a new section of questions, and whenever the person introduces a new topic (e.g., "Tell me why you have come here today," or "What brings you to the clinic or hospital?").

Closed or Direct Questions

Closed or **direct questions** ask for specific information. They elicit a short one- or two-word answer, a "yes" or "no," or a forced choice. Use direct questions after the patient's opening narrative to fill in any details that the patient left out. In addition, use direct questions when you need many specific facts, such as when asking about past health problems or during the review of systems.

Responses: Assisting the Narrative

As the patient talks, your role is to encourage free expression, but not let the patient digress. The following responses help you gather data without cutting the person off.

Facilitation. These responses—also called *general leads*—encourage the patient to say more, to continue with the story (e.g., "Mmm-hmm," "Go on," "Please continue," "Uh-huh," or simply nodding). Maintaining eye contact, shifting forward in your seat with increased attention, or using hand gestures also encourages the patient to continue talking.

Silence. Your silent attentiveness communicates to patients that they have time to think, to organize what they wish to say without interruption. Also, silence gives you a chance to observe patients unobtrusively and to note nonverbal cues.

Reflection. This response echoes the patient's words. Reflection is repeating part of what the patient has just said. It focuses further attention on a specific phrase and helps the patient continue to answer.

Empathy. An empathic response relays recognition of a feeling, puts it into words, and allows the expression of it. When the empathic response is used, the patient feels accepted and can deal with the feeling openly. Empathic responses include saying, "This must be very hard for you" and just placing your hand on the patient's arm.

Clarification. Seek clarification when the patient's word choice is ambiguous or confusing (e.g., "Tell me what you mean by 'tired blood.'") Clarification may also focus on a discrepancy ("You say it doesn't hurt, but when I touch you here, you grimace."), or the patient's affect ("You *look* sad." or "You *sound* angry.").

Interpretation. An interpretive response is based on your inferences or conclusions. It links events, makes associations, or implies cause ("It seems that every time you feel the stomach pain, you have had some kind of stress in your life.").

Explanation. With these statements, you give the patient information. You share factual and objective data. This information may be for orientation to the health care setting ("Your dinner comes at 5:30 P.M."), or it may be to explain cause ("The reason you cannot eat or drink before your blood test is that the food will affect the test results, and we would like to get as accurate a result as possible.").

Summary. This is a final review of your understanding of what the patient has said. In summarizing, you condense the facts and present a survey of how you perceive the patient's health problem or need.

CLOSING THE INTERVIEW

The session should end gracefully. To ease into the closing, ask the patient questions such as, "Is there anything else you would like to mention?" This gives the patient the final opportunity for self-expression. This is a good time to give your summary or recapitulation of what you have learned during the interview. It should include positive health aspects, any health issues or priorities that have been identified, any plans for action, or an explanation of the subsequent physical examination. As you part from patients, thank them for the time spent and for their participation.

TEN TRAPS OF INTERVIEWING

Nonproductive, defeating verbal messages are messages that restrict the patient's response. They are obstacles to obtaining accurate, complete data and to establishing rapport.

1. Providing False Assurance or Reassurance. A statement such as, "Now don't worry; I'm sure you will be all right" is a "courage builder" that relieves *your* anxiety and gives you the false sense of having provided comfort. For patients, however, it actually closes off communication. It trivializes their anxiety and effectively denies any further talk of it.

2. Giving Unwanted Advice. A patient describes a problem to you, ending with, "What would you do?" If you answer, "If I were you, I'd... ," you have shifted the accountability for decision making from the patient to you. The patient has not worked out his or her own solution by considering available options and has learned nothing about himself or herself.

3. Using Authority. "Your doctor/ nurse knows best" is a response that promotes dependency and inferiority.

4. Using Avoidance Language. People use euphemisms such as "passed on" to avoid reality or to hide their feelings.

5. Engaging in Distancing. Distancing is the use of impersonal speech to put space between a threat and the self (e.g., "There is a blockage in the artery.").

6. Overusing Professional Jargon or Casual Language. Use of jargon sounds exclusionary and paternalistic. You need to adjust your vocabulary to the patient but avoid sounding condescending or too medicalized.

7. Using Leading or Biased Questions. Asking a question such as "You don't smoke, do you?" implies that one answer is "better" than another.

8. Talking Too Much. Some examiners positively associate helpfulness with verbal productivity. These examiners leave thinking they have met the patient's needs. Just the opposite is true.

9. Interrupting. Often, when you think you know what the patient will say, you interrupt and cut the patient off.

10. Using "Why" Questions. The adult's use of "why" questions (such as "Why were you so late for your appointment?") implies blame and condemnation; it puts the patient on the defensive.

Nonverbal Skills

Nonverbal messages that are productive and enhancing to the relationship are those that show attentiveness and unconditional acceptance. Defeating, nonproductive nonverbal behaviours are those of inattentiveness, authority, and superiority (Table 1.1).

TABLE 1.1	Nonverbal Behaviours of the Interviewer
Positive	Negative
Professional appearance is appropriate to the context	Appearance objectionable to patient
Equal-status seating	Standing
Close proximity to patient	Sitting behind desk, far away, turned away
Relaxed open posture	Tense posture
Leaning slightly toward patient	Slouched back
Occasional facilitation gestures	Critical or distracting gestures: pointing finger, clenched fist, finger tapping, foot swinging, looking at watch
Facial animation, interest	Bland expression, yawning, tight mouth
Appropriate smiling	Frowning, lip-biting
Appropriate eye contact	Shifty; avoiding eye contact; focusing on notes, computer screen, iPad, etc.
Moderate tone of voice	Strident, high-pitched tone
Moderate rate of speech	Rate too slow or too fast
Appropriate use and consent of touch, depending on the context	Too frequent or inappropriate touch; touch without consent of patient and/or patient's caregiver

HEALTH HISTORY: ADULTS

Biographical Data

This information includes the patient's name, address, and phone number, age and birthdate, birthplace, other recent countries of residence, sex, gender, relationship status, and usual and current occupation.

Source of History

The history may be provided by the patient, a parent, or by a substitute (such as a relative or friend).

Reason for Seeking Care

This is a brief spontaneous statement in the patient's own words that describes the reason for the visit.

Current Health or History of Current Illness

For the well patient, current health is a short statement about the general state of health.

For the ill patient, this section is a chronological record of the reason for seeking care, from the time the symptom first started until now. Your final summary of any symptom the patient has should include these critical characteristics, organized into the mnemonic **PQRSTU** to help remember all the points.

P (provocative or palliative) "What brings it on? What were you doing when you first noticed it? What makes it better? Worse?"

Q (quality or quantity) "How does it look, feel, sound? How intense or severe is it?"

R (region or radiation) "Where is it? Does it spread anywhere?"

S (severity scale) "How bad is it (on a scale of 1 to 10)? Is it getting better, worse, or staying the same?"

T (timing) "Exactly when did it first occur?" (onset); "How long did it last?" (duration); "How often does it occur?" (frequency)

U (understand patient's perception of the problem): "What do you think it means?"

Past Health History

Childhood Illnesses. Measles, mumps, rubella, chicken pox, pertussis, streptococcal infection ("strep throat"), rheumatic fever, scarlet fever, and poliomyelitis.

Accidents or Injuries. Auto accidents, fractures, penetrating wounds, head injuries (especially if associated with unconsciousness), and burns.

Serious or Chronic Illnesses. Diabetes, hypertension, heart disease, sickle cell disease, cancer, and seizure disorder.

Hospitalizations. Cause, name of the hospital, how the condition was treated, how long the patient was hospitalized, and name of the treating physician.

Operations. Type of surgery, date of surgery, name of the surgeon, name of the hospital, and how the patient recovered.

Obstetrical History. The number of pregnancies (gravidity, or *grav*), number of deliveries in which the fetus reached full term *(term)*, number of preterm deliveries *(preterm)*, number of incomplete pregnancies or abortions *(ab)*, and number of living children *(living)*. This is recorded as: "Grav___Term___Preterm___Ab___ Living___".

Immunizations. Depending on the patient's age group, ask whether the patient has received measles-mumps-rubella, polio, diphtheria-pertussis-tetanus, hepatitis B, human papillomavirus, *Haemophilus influenzae* type b, and pneumococcal vaccine. Note the dates of the most recent tetanus immunization, most recent tuberculosis skin test, and most recent influenza shot.

Most Recent Examination Date. The most recent physical, dental, vision, hearing, electrocardiographic, and chest radiographic examinations.

Allergies. Medication, food, or contact agent. Note reaction.

Current Medications. All prescription and over-the-counter medications, including vitamins and other supplements, birth control pills, aspirin, and antacids.

Family Health History

The age and health, or the age at and cause of death of blood relatives, such as parents or other primary caregivers, grandparents, and siblings. The age and health of spouse and children. Specifically, any family history of heart disease, high blood pressure, stroke, diabetes, blood disorders, cancer, sickle cell disease, arthritis, allergies, obesity, alcoholism, mental health issues or illness, seizure disorder, kidney disease, or tuberculosis. Construct a family tree, or genogram, to show this information clearly and concisely (Fig. 1.1).

Review of Systems

General Overall Health State. Ask how the patient feels overall in terms of physical, mental, emotional, and spiritual health. Current weight (gain or loss, period of time, by diet or other factors), fatigue, weakness or malaise, fever, chills, and sweats or night sweats.

Skin, Hair, and Nails. History of skin disease (eczema, psoriasis, hives), pigment or colour change, change in mole, excessive dryness or moisture, pruritus, excessive bruising, and rash or lesion. Document recent loss and change in texture. For nails, note change in shape, colour, or brittleness.

Health Promotion. Ask what the patient is doing to stay healthy and for prevention. Amount of sun exposure and use of sunscreen and use of appropriate footwear to prevent foot sores (for a patient with diabetes).

<u>**Drawing Your Family Tree**</u>
- Make a list of all of your family members.
- Use this sample family tree as a guide to draw your own family tree.
- Write your name at the top of your paper and date you drew your family tree.
- In place of the words father, mother, etc., write the names of your family members.
- When possible, draw your brothers and sisters and your parents' brothers and sisters starting from oldest to youngest, going from left to right across the paper.
- If dates of birth or ages are not known, then estimate or guess ("50s," "late 60s").

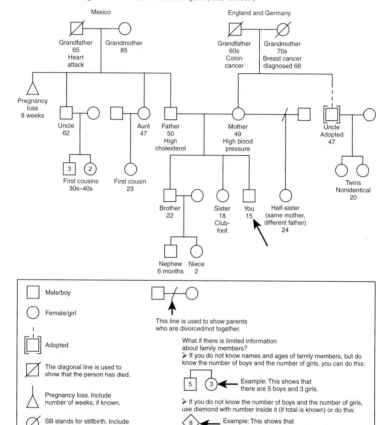

1.1 Genogram or family tree.

Head. Unusually frequent or severe headache, any head injury, dizziness (syncope), or vertigo.

Health Promotion. Depending on the patient's age, geographical location, and social–personal circumstances, ask, for example, about use of protective gear during sports activities.

Eyes. Difficulty with vision (decreased acuity, blurring, blind spots), eye pain, diplopia (double vision), redness or swelling, watering or discharge, glaucoma, or cataracts.

Health Promotion. Glasses or contact lens wear, most recent vision check or glaucoma test, how the patient copes with loss of vision (if any).

Ears. Earaches, infections, discharge and its characteristics, tinnitus, or vertigo.

Health Promotion. Hearing loss, hearing aid use, how loss affects daily life, exposure to environmental noise, use of earplugs or other noise-reducing devices, and method of cleaning ears.

Nose and Sinuses. Discharge and its characteristics, unusually frequent or severe colds, any sinus pain, nasal obstruction, nosebleeds, allergies or hay fever, or change in sense of smell.

Mouth and Throat. Mouth pain, frequent sore throat, bleeding gums, toothache, lesion in mouth or on tongue, dysphagia, hoarseness or voice change, tonsillectomy, or altered taste.

Health Promotion. Pattern of daily dental care, use of prosthesis (dentures, bridge), and most recent dental checkup.

Neck. Pain, limitation of motion, lumps or swelling, enlarged or tender nodes, or goitre.

Breast. Pain, lump, nipple discharge, rash, breast disease, and any surgery on the breasts.

Health Promotion. Date of most recent mammogram, performance of breast self-examination.

Axilla. Tenderness, lump or swelling, or rash.

Respiratory System. History of lung diseases (asthma, emphysema, bronchitis, pneumonia, tuberculosis), chest pain with breathing, wheezing or noisy breathing, shortness of breath, how much activity produces shortness of breath, cough, sputum (colour, amount), hemoptysis, and toxin or pollution exposure.

Health Promotion. Date of most recent chest X-ray study.

Cardiovascular System. Precordial or retrosternal pain, palpitation, cyanosis, dyspnea on exertion (specify amount of exertion that triggers dyspnea), orthopnea, paroxysmal nocturnal dyspnea, nocturia, edema, and history of heart murmur, hypertension, coronary artery disease, and anemia.

Health Promotion. Date of most recent electrocardiogram or other tests of heart function.

Peripheral Vascular System. Coldness, numbness and tingling, swelling of legs (time of day and activity), discoloration in hands or feet (bluish red, pallor, mottling, associated with position, especially around feet and ankles), varicose veins or complications, intermittent claudication, thrombophlebitis, and ulcers.

Health Promotion. Amount of long-term sitting or standing, habit of crossing legs at the knees, use of support hose.

Gastro-intestinal System. Appetite, food intolerance, dysphagia, heartburn, indigestion, pain (associated with eating), other abdominal pain, pyrosis (esophageal and stomach burning sensation with sour eructation), nausea and vomiting (character), vomiting blood, history of abdominal disease (ulcer, liver or gallbladder, jaundice, appendicitis, colitis), flatulence, frequency of bowel movements (any recent change), stool characteristics, constipation or diarrhea, black stools, rectal bleeding, and rectal conditions (hemorrhoids, fistula).

Health Promotion. Use of antacids or laxatives. (Alternatively, diet history can be described in this section.)

Urinary System. Frequency or urgency, nocturia (the number of times the patient awakens at night to urinate; recent change), dysuria, polyuria, oliguria, hesitancy or straining, narrowed stream, urine colour (cloudy or presence of hematuria), incontinence, history of urinary disease (kidney disease, kidney stones, urinary tract infections, prostate disease), and pain in flank, groin, suprapubic region, or lower back.

Health Promotion. Measures to avoid or treat urinary tract infections, use of Kegel exercises after childbirth.

Male Genital System. Penile or testicular pain, sores or lesions, penile discharge, lumps, or hernia.

Health Promotion. Performance of testicular self-examination and frequency.

Female Genital System. Menstrual history (age at menarche, most recent menstrual period, cycle and duration, any amenorrhea or menorrhagia, premenstrual pain or dysmenorrhea, intermenstrual spotting), vaginal itching, discharge and its characteristics, age at menopause, menopausal signs or symptoms, and postmenopausal bleeding.

Health Promotion. Most recent gynecological checkup and most recent Papanicolaou (Pap) test.

Sexual Health. Current sexual activity (in a relationship involving intercourse), level of sexual satisfaction of patient and partner, dyspareunia (for a female patient), changes in erection or ejaculation (for a male patient), use of contraceptive and satisfaction with it, any known or suspected contact with a partner who has a sexually transmitted infection (STI; e.g., gonorrhea, herpes, chlamydia, venereal warts, human immunodeficiency virus [HIV] infection or acquired immune deficiency syndrome [AIDS], or syphilis).

Musculo-skeletal System. History of arthritis or gout. Joint pain, stiffness, swelling (location, migratory nature), deformity, limitation of motion, or noise with joint motion. Muscle pain, cramps, weakness, gait problems, or problems with coordinated activities. Back pain (location and radiation to extremities), stiffness, limitation of motion, or history of back pain or disc disease.

Health Promotion. Distance walked per day, effect of limited range of motion on daily activities such as grooming, eating, toileting, or dressing, and use of mobility aids. For older adults, ask about fall prevention strategies.

Neurological System. History of seizure disorder, stroke, fainting, or blackouts. In motor function, weakness, tic or tremor, paralysis, or coordination problems. In sensory function, numbness and tingling (paresthesia). In cognitive function, memory disorder (recent or distant, disorientation). In mental status, nervousness, mood change, depression, or history of mental health dysfunction or hallucinations.

Health Promotion. Data about interpersonal relationships and coping patterns can be placed in this section.

Hematological System. Bleeding tendency of skin or mucous membranes, excessive bruising, lymph node swelling, exposure to toxic agents or radiation, blood transfusion and reactions.

Endocrine System. History of diabetes or diabetic symptoms (polyuria, polydipsia, polyphagia), history of thyroid disease, intolerance to heat and cold, change in skin pigmentation or texture, excessive sweating, relationship between appetite and weight, abnormal hair distribution, nervousness, tremors, and need for hormone therapy.

Health Promotion. Depending on a diabetic patient's health history, ask about use of appropriate footwear to prevent foot sores or ulcers.

Functional Assessment (Including Activities of Daily Living)

In a functional assessment, you measure a patient's self-care ability in the areas of physical health or absence of illness; activities of daily living (ADLs), such as bathing, dressing, toileting, eating, and walking; instrumental activities of daily living (IADLs), which are activities needed for independent living, such as housekeeping, shopping, cooking, doing laundry, using the telephone, and managing finances; nutrition; social relationships and resources; self-concept and coping; and home environment. These questions provide data on the lifestyle and type of living environment to which the patient is accustomed.

Self-Concept, Self-Esteem. Education level (last grade completed, other significant training), financial status (income adequate and health or social concerns), and value–belief system (religious practices and perception of personal strengths).

Activity and Mobility. Obtain a daily profile that reflects usual daily activities. Ask, "Tell me how you spend a typical day." Ability to perform ADLs—independent or needs assistance. Use of wheelchair, prostheses, or mobility aids. Leisure activities enjoyed and exercise pattern (type, amount per day or week, method of warm-up session, method of monitoring the body's response to exercise).

Sleep and Rest. Sleep patterns, daytime naps, any sleep aids used.

Nutrition and Elimination. All food and beverages taken over the past 24 hours. Ask, "Is that menu typical of most days?" Eating habits and current appetite. Ask, "Who buys food and prepares food?"; "Are your finances adequate for food?"; and "Who is present at mealtimes?" Food allergy or intolerance. Daily intake of caffeine (coffee, tea, cola drinks).

Usual pattern of bowel elimination and urinating, problems with mobility or transfer in toileting, continence, use of laxatives.

Interpersonal Relationships and Resources. Social roles. Ask, "How would you describe your role in the family?" and "How would you say you get along with family, friends, and coworkers?" Support systems composed of family and significant others. Ask, "To whom could you go for support with a problem at work, a health problem, or a personal problem?" Contact with spouse, siblings, parents, children, chosen family, friends, organizations, and the workplace. Ask, "Is time spent alone pleasurable and relaxing, or is it isolating?"

Spiritual Resources. Use faith, influence, community, and address (**FICA**) questions to incorporate the patient's spiritual values into the health history.

Coping and Stress Management. Life stresses in the past year, any change in living situation or any current stress, and any methods for dealing with stress.

Personal Habits. Smoking history. Ask about smoking patterns in a nonjudgemental way. "Do you smoke?"; "At what age did you start?"; "How many packs do you smoke per day?"; and "How many years have you smoked?"

Alcohol. Convey acceptance and a nonjudgemental attitude when discussing alcohol patterns. "Do you drink alcohol?"; and "How much do you drink each day (or week)?"

Substance use. Ask about substance use in effective, respectful ways. "Have you ever tried any drugs such as marijuana, cocaine, amphetamines, or barbiturates?"; "How often do you use these drugs?"; and "How has usage affected your work, social relationships, family, and finances?"

Environmental Hazards. Housing and neighbourhood (live alone, know neighbours, safety of area, adequate heat and utilities, access to transportation, involved in community services). Environmental health (hazards in workplace, hazards at home, excessive screen use, use of seatbelts and helmets, geographical or occupational exposures, travel, or residence in other countries).

Intimate Partner Violence. Ask nonjudgemental, open-ended questions. "How are things at home (or at school or work)?"; "How are things at home affecting your health?"; and "Is your home (or work or school) environment safe?" Patients may not recognize their situations as abusive, or they may be reluctant to discuss their situation because of guilt, fear, or shame. Follow each patient's lead to inquire more specifically.

Occupational Health. Ask the patient to describe their employment situation; the patient may or may not have a clearly identifiable job. "Have you ever worked with any health hazard, such as asbestos, inhalants, chemicals, and repetitive motion?"; "Do you wear or use any protective equipment?"; "Are any work programs in place to monitor your exposure?"; "Are you aware of any health problems now that may be related to work exposure?"; and "What do you like or dislike about your work?"

Perception of Health

Ask the patient questions such as "What does it mean to you to be healthy? How do you define health?"; "How do you view your situation now?"; "What are your concerns?"; "What do you think will happen in the future?"; "What are your health goals?"; and "What do you expect from us as nurses, nurse practitioners, physicians, or other health care providers?"

For more information on the health history of infants and children, older adults, and cultural assessment, see Chapter 5 in Jarvis, *Physical Examination & Health Assessment,* 3rd Canadian edition, pages 70.

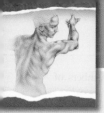

CHAPTER 2

Mental Health Assessment

Mental status is a person's emotional and cognitive functioning. Optimal functioning aims toward simultaneous life satisfaction in work, in caring relationships, and within the self.

Mental status cannot be scrutinized directly like the characteristics of skin or heart sounds. Its functioning is *inferred* through assessment of an individual's behaviours and mental health functions:

Appearance: General presentation to others.

Consciousness: Being aware of one's feelings, thoughts, and environment.

Speech: Using language and the voice to communicate one's thoughts and feelings.

Mood and affect: Expressing the prevailing feelings through mood (a sustained emotion that the patient is experiencing) and affect (a display of feelings or state of mind).

Orientation: Awareness of the objective world in relation to the self.

Attention and concentration: The power to direct thinking toward an object or topic with the ability to focus on one specific thing without being distracted by other competing stimuli.

Memory: The ability to set down and store experiences and perceptions for later recall; *immediate* memory involves on-the-spot recall, *recent* memory evokes day-to-day events, and *remote* memory includes years' worth of experiences.

Comprehension and abstract reasoning: Pondering a deeper meaning beyond the concrete and literal.

Thought process: The way a person thinks; the logical train of thought.

Thought content: What the person thinks; specific ideas, beliefs, the use of words.

Perception: An awareness of objects through the five senses.

Insight: Awareness of the reality of the situation.

Judgement: Ability to choose a logical course of action.

THE MENTAL STATUS EXAMINATION

The full mental status examination is a systematic check of emotional and cognitive functioning, and is an essential part of the mental health assessment. Most of this information can be obtained indirectly while conducting a general health assessment. During that time, keep in mind the four main domains of mental status assessment:

Appearance
Behaviour
Cognition
Thought processes

In every mental health assessment, note the following factors that could affect your interpretation:
• Any known illnesses or health problems, such as problematic alcohol use or chronic renal disease.

11

- Current medications, the adverse effects of which may cause confusion or depression.
- The usual educational and behavioural level; note that factor as the normal baseline, and do not expect performance on the mental health assessment to exceed it.
- Responses to personal history questions, indicating current stress, social interaction patterns, sleep habits, and drug and alcohol use.

Appearance

Posture. *Posture* is erect, and *position* is relaxed.

Body Movements. *Body movements* are voluntary, deliberate, coordinated, and smooth and even.

Dress. *Dress* is appropriate for setting, season, age, gender, and social group. Clothing fits and is put on appropriately.

Grooming and Hygiene. The patient is clean and well groomed; hair is neat and clean; women have moderate or no makeup; men are shaved or beard or moustache is well-groomed. Nails are clean (though some jobs leave nails chronically dirty). Use care in interpreting clothing that is dishevelled, bizarre, or in poor repair; piercings; and tattoos, because these sometimes reflect the person's economic status or a deliberate fashion trend (especially among adolescents).

Behaviour

Level of Consciousness. The patient is awake, alert, and aware of stimuli from the environment and within the self and responds appropriately to stimuli (Table 2.1).

Facial Expression. The expression is appropriate to the situation and changes appropriately with the topic. There is comfortable eye contact unless precluded by cultural

norm, for example, for members of some Aboriginal cultures.

Speech. Judge the *quality* of speech by noting that the patient makes laryngeal sounds effortlessly and makes conversation appropriately. Note whether the voice is raised or muffled, whether the replies to questions are one-word or elaborative, and how fast or slow the patient speaks.

The *pace* of the conversation is moderate, and stream of talking is fluent.

Articulation (ability to form words) is clear and understandable.

Word choice is effortless and appropriate to educational level. The patient completes sentences, occasionally pausing to think.

Mood and Affect. Judge this by body language and facial expression and by asking the answer to the direct question "How do you feel today?" or "How do you feel most days?" Ask about the length of a particular mood, whether the mood has been reactive or not, and whether the mood has been stable or unstable. The affect (expression) should be appropriate to the mood and change appropriately with topics.

Cognitive Functions

Orientation. You can discern orientation through the course of the interview. Assess:

Time: day of week, date, year, season
Place: where person lives, present location, type of building, names of city and province
Person: who examiner is, type of worker
Self: person's own name, age

Many hospitalized patients normally have trouble with the exact date but are fully oriented on the remaining items.

TABLE 2.1	Levels of Consciousness

The terms below are commonly used in clinical practice.
To increase clarity, also record:

1. The level of stimulus used, ranging progressively from:
   - Name called in normal tone of voice
   - Name called in loud voice
   - Light touch on person's arm
   - Vigorous shake of shoulder
   - Pain applied
2. The patient's response:
   - Amount and quality of movement
   - Presence and coherence of speech
   - Opens eyes and makes eye contact
3. What the person does on cessation of your stimulus:

   Alert
   Awake or readily aroused, oriented, fully aware of external and internal stimuli and responds appropriately, conducts meaningful interpersonal interactions

   Lethargic (or Somnolent)
   Not fully alert, drifts off to sleep when not stimulated; can be aroused to name when called in normal voice but looks drowsy; responds appropriately to questions or commands, but thinking seems slow and fuzzy; inattentive, loses train of thought, spontaneous movements are decreased

   Obtunded
   (Transitional state between lethargy and stupor)
   Sleeps most of time, difficult to arouse; needs loud shout or vigorous shake, acts confused when aroused, converses in monosyllables, speech may be mumbled and incoherent, requires constant stimulation for even marginal cooperation

   Stupor or Semicoma
   Spontaneously unconscious, responds only to persistent and vigorous shake or pain; has appropriate motor response (i.e., withdraws hand to avoid pain); otherwise can only groan, mumble, or move restlessly; reflex activity persists

   Coma
   Completely unconscious, no response to pain or to any external or internal stimuli (e.g., when suctioned, does not try to push the catheter away); in light coma, has some reflex activity but not purposeful movement; in deep coma, has no motor response

   Acute Confusional State (Delirium)
   Clouding of consciousness (dulled cognition, impaired alertness); inattentive; incoherent conversation; impaired recent memory and confabulatory for recent events; often agitated and having visual hallucinations; disoriented, with confusion worse at night when environmental stimuli are decreased

Adapted from Porth, C. (2007). *Essentials of pathophysiology: Concepts of altered health states* (p. 835). Hagerstown, MD: Lippincott Williams & Wilkins.

Attention Span. Check the patient's ability to concentrate by noting whether the patient completes a thought without wandering. Note any distractibility or difficulty attending to you. An alternative approach is to give a series of directions to follow in a correct sequence of behaviours, such as "Please put this label on your keys, place the keys into the brown envelope, and give the envelope to the clerk for safe keeping during your admission." Be aware that attention span commonly is impaired in people who experience anxiety, fatigue, drug intoxication, or attention-deficit/hyperactivity disorder.

Immediate Memory. Assess immediate memory by asking the patient to recall a statement you just made.

Recent Memory. Assess recent memory in the context of the interview by the 24-hour diet recall or asking what time the patient arrived at the agency. Ask verifiable questions to screen for the occasional person who confabulates (makes up) answers to fill in the gaps of memory loss.

Remote Memory. In the context of the interview, ask the patient about verifiable past events; for example, ask to describe historic events that are relevant for the patient.

Insight and Judgement. To assess judgement in the context of the interview, note what the person says about job plans and social or family obligations; plans for the future; and capacity for violent or suicidal behaviour. Further assess insight by asking patients to describe their rationale for personal health care and how they decided about whether to comply with prescribed health regimens. The patient's actions and decisions should be realistic.

Thought Processes, Thought Content, and Perceptions

Thought Processes. Ask yourself, "Does this person make sense? Can I follow what the person is saying?" The *way* a patient thinks should be logical, goal directed, coherent, and relevant. The patient should complete a thought.

Thought Content. *What* the patient says should be consistent and logical. Ask questions to identify any obsessions or compulsions (e.g., "Do you perform specific actions to reduce certain thoughts?"), fears (such

as fear of animals, needles, heights, etc.), or delusions (e.g., "Do you have any thoughts that other people think are strange?").

Perceptions. The patient should be consistently aware of reality, and his or her perceptions should be congruent with yours. Ask the following:

- "How do people treat you?"
- "Do you feel as if you are being watched, followed, or controlled?"
- "Is your imagination very active?"
- "Have you heard your name when you're alone?"

If the responses to these questions suggest that a person is experiencing hallucinations, ask questions such as, "Do you ever hear voices when no one else is around?"

Screen for Suicidal Thoughts. While it is difficult to question patients about possible suicidal wishes, the risk is far greater if you skip these questions; you may be the only health care provider to detect clues of suicide risk. When the patient expresses feelings of sadness, hopelessness, despair, or grief, assess any possible risk that the patient will cause physical harm to himself or herself. Begin with more general questions; if you hear affirmative answers, continue with more specific questions:

"Have you ever felt so blue you thought of hurting yourself?"

"Do you feel like hurting yourself now?"

"Do you have a plan to hurt yourself?"

"What would happen if you were dead?"

"How would other people react if you were dead?"

You are responsible for encouraging the patient to talk about suicidal thoughts and for obtaining immediate help. Although you cannot always prevent a suicide, you can often buy time so that the patient can be helped to find an alternative solution to problems.

Supplemental Mental Status Examination

The Mini-Cog test and the Addenbrooke's Cognitive Examination-Revised (ACE-R) are the best alternative screening tests for dementia, and the Montreal Cognitive Assessment (MoCA) (Fig. 2.1) is the best alternative for mild cognitive impairment (Tsoi et al., 2015). The Mini-Cog takes 3 minutes to administer; it can

increase detection of cognitive impairment in older adults. It is useful in detecting Alzheimer's and related dementia. It can be used effectively after brief training in both health care and community settings. It consists of two components, a three-item recall test for memory, and a simply scored clock drawing test. As a screening test, however, it does not substitute for a complete diagnostic workup (Tsoi et al., 2015).

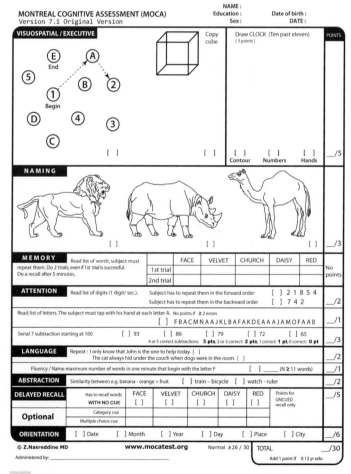

2.1 Montreal Cognitive Assessment. *(Copyright Z. Nasreddine, MD. Reproduced with permission. Copies are available at www.mocatest.org.)*

The Rowland Universal Dementia Assessment Scale (RUDAS), a multi-cultural cognitive assessment scale, is a short cognitive screening instrument designed to minimize the effects of cultural learning and language diversity on the assessment of baseline cognitive performance. It is recommended that the RUDAS respondent communicate in the language they are most competent and comfortable with. Prior to administrating the RUDAS, the provider should read the instructions carefully (Storey et al., 2004). For more information on abnormalities of mood and affect, delirium and dementia, substance use disorders, schizophrenia, mood disorders, and anxiety disorders, see Chapter 6 in Jarvis: *Physical Examination and Health Assessment,* 3rd Canadian edition, pages 78–109.

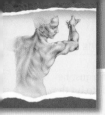

Assessment Techniques and the Clinical Setting

ASSESSMENT TECHNIQUES

The skills requisite for the physical examination are **inspection**, **palpation**, **percussion**, and **auscultation**. The skills are performed one at a time and in this order.

Inspection

Inspection is concentrated watching. It is close, careful scrutiny, first of the individual patient as a whole and then of each body system. Inspection begins the moment you first meet the patient and develop a "general survey." (Specific data to consider for the general survey are described in the following chapter.) As you proceed through the examination, start the assessment of each body system with inspection.

Learn to use each patient as his or her own control by comparing the right and left sides of the body. The two sides are nearly symmetrical. Inspection requires good lighting, adequate exposure, and occasional use of certain instruments (otoscope, ophthalmoscope, penlight, nasal and vaginal specula) to enlarge your view.

Palpation

Palpation follows and often confirms points you noted during inspection. In palpation, you apply your sense of touch to assess texture, temperature, moisture, and organ location and size, as well as any swelling, vibration or pulsation, rigidity or spasticity,

crepitation, presence of lumps or masses, and presence of tenderness or pain. Different parts of your hands are best suited for assessing different factors:

- Fingertips: Best for fine tactile discrimination such as skin texture, swelling, pulsation, and determining presence of lumps
- A grasping action between the fingers and thumb: To detect the position, shape, and consistency of an organ or mass
- The dorsa (backs) of hands and fingers: Best for determining temperature because the skin is thinner on the dorsa than on the palms
- Base of fingers (metacarpophalangeal joints) or ulnar surface of the hand: Best for vibration

Your palpation technique should be slow and systematic. Warm your hands by kneading them together or holding them under warm water. Identify any tender areas, and palpate them last.

Start with light palpation, using the pads of your fingertips to detect surface characteristics and to accustom the patient to being touched.

When deep palpation is needed (as for abdominal contents), intermittent pressure is better than one long, continuous palpation. Avoid deep palpation in situations in which it could cause internal injury or pain.

Bimanual palpation requires the use of both of your hands to envelop or detect certain body parts or organs—such as the kidneys, uterus, or adnexa—for more precise delimitation.

Percussion

Percussion is tapping the person's skin with short, sharp strokes to assess underlying structures. The strokes yield a palpable vibration and a characteristic sound that depicts the location, size, and density of the underlying organ.

The Stationary Hand. Hyperextend the middle finger (sometimes called the *pleximeter*) of your nondominant hand and place its distal joint firmly against the patient's skin. Avoid the patient's ribs and scapulae; percussing over a bone yields no data because it always sounds "dull." Lift the rest of the stationary hand off the patient's skin (Fig. 3.1); otherwise the stationary hand will dampen the produced vibrations, just as a drummer uses the hand to halt a drum roll.

The Striking Hand. Use the middle finger of your dominant hand as the *striking finger* (the *plexor*). Hold your forearm close to the patient's skin surface, with your upper arm and shoulder steady. The action is all in the wrist, and it must be relaxed. Spread your fingers, flick your wrist, and bounce your middle finger off

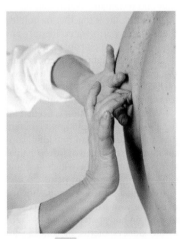

3.1 Percussion.

the stationary finger. Aim for just behind the nail bed; the goal is to hit the portion of the finger that is pushing the hardest into the patient's skin surface. Flex the striking finger so that its tip, not the finger pad, makes contact. It hits directly at right angles to the stationary finger.

- Percuss two times in this location, using even, staccato blows. Lift the striking finger off quickly; a resting finger dampens vibrations. Then move to a new body location and repeat, keeping your technique even (Table 3.1).

Auscultation

Auscultation is listening to sounds produced by parts of the body, such as the heart and blood vessels, the lungs, and the abdomen, through a **stethoscope.**

Choose a stethoscope with two end pieces: a diaphragm and a bell. You use the **diaphragm** most often because its flat edge is best for hearing high-pitched sounds: breath, bowel, and normal heart sounds. Hold the diaphragm against the patient's skin firmly enough to leave a slight ring afterward.

The **bell** endpiece has a deep, hollow, cuplike shape. It is best for soft, low-pitched sounds such as extra heart sounds or murmurs. Hold it lightly against the patient's skin, just enough that it forms a perfect seal. Pressing any harder causes the patient's skin to act as a diaphragm, obliterating the low-pitched sounds.

Some newer stethoscopes have one end piece with a "tunable diaphragm." This enables you to listen to both low- and high-frequency sounds without rotation of the endpiece.

SETTING: CONTEXT OF CARE

- The examination room should be warm and comfortable, quiet, private, and well-lit.

TABLE 3.1	Characteristics of Percussion Notes				
Type	Amplitude	Pitch	Quality	Duration	Sample Location
Resonant	Medium-loud	Low	Clear, hollow	Moderate	Over normal lung tissue
Hyperresonant	Louder	Lower	Booming	Longer	Normal finding over a child's lung. Abnormal finding in an adult over lungs with increased amount of air, as in emphysema
Tympany	Loud	High	Musical and drumlike (like the kettle drum)	Sustained longest	Over air-filled viscus, such as the stomach or the intestine
Dull	Soft	High	Muffled thud	Short	Relatively dense organ such as liver or spleen
Flat	Very soft	High	An instant stop of sound; absolute dullness	Very short	When no air is present, over thigh muscles, bone, or tumour

- Ensure the environment is safe by performing an **environmental scan** of the examination area (note devices attached to the patient; look for obvious environmental or biomedical hazards (such as liquid on the floor); consider any patient safety concerns (such as bedside rails being down); ensure that necessary equipment for the assessment is in place).
- When possible, stop or minimize any distracting noises.
- Discourage interruptions.
- Lighting with natural daylight is best, although artificial light from two sources suffices and prevents shadows.
- Position a wall-mounted or gooseneck stand lamp for high-intensity lighting.
- Position the patient so that both sides of their body are easily accessible.
- The examination or bedside table should be at a height at which you can stand without stooping and should be equipped to raise the person's head up to 45 degrees.
- A roll-up stool is used for the sections of the examination for which you must be sitting.
- A bedside stand, table, or flat surface is needed to lay out all your equipment.

EQUIPMENT

Have all your equipment within easy reach and laid out in an organized manner. The following items are usually needed for a screening physical examination:

- Platform scale with height attachment
- Sphygmomanometer (blood pressure monitor)
- Stethoscope with bell and diaphragm endpieces
- Thermometer
- Data collection device (pen and paper, computer)
- Pulse oximeter (in hospital or clinic setting)
- Flashlight or penlight
- Otoscope/ophthalmoscope
- Nasal speculum (if a short, broad speculum is not included with the otoscope)
- Tuning fork
- Tongue depressor
- Pocket vision screener
- Skin-marking pen
- Flexible tape measure and ruler marked in centimetres
- Reflex hammer
- Sharp object (split tongue blade)
- Cotton balls
- Clean gloves
- Hand sanitizer or access to a sink
- Lubricant
- Watch or timing device

A CLEAN FIELD

Designate "clean" and "used" areas for handling of your equipment. Distinguish the clean area by one or two disposable paper towels. On the towels, place all the new, newly cleaned, or newly alcohol-swabbed equipment that you will use on the current patient (e.g., your stethoscope endpieces, the reflex hammer, the ruler).

Equipment that is used frequently on many patients can become a common vehicle for transmission of infection. As you proceed through the examination, pick up each piece of equipment from the clean area and, after use on the patient, place it in the used area, or (as in the case of tongue blades and gloves) throw it directly into the garbage.

A SAFER ENVIRONMENT

Take all steps to avoid any possible transmission of infection between patients or between patient and examiner. The single most important step to decrease risk of microorganism transmission is to first establish, through a point-of-care risk assessment (PCRA), what the likelihood of exposure is and then determine the appropriate actions. The most effective primary intervention continues to be to wash your hands promptly and thoroughly: (a) **before** initial patient/patient environmental contact; (b) **before** aseptic procedures; (c) **after** contact with blood, body fluids, secretions, and excretions; (d) **after** contact with any equipment contaminated with body fluids; and (e) **after** removing gloves. Using alcohol-based hand rubs takes less time than soap-and-water handwashing; it also kills more organisms more quickly and is less damaging to the skin because of emollients added to the product. Use the mechanical action of soap-and-water handwashing when hands are visibly soiled and when patients are infected with spore-forming organisms.

Wear gloves when the potential exists for contact with any body fluids (e.g., blood, mucous membranes, body fluids, drainage, and open skin lesions). However, wearing gloves is *not* a protective substitute for washing hands because gloves may have undetectable holes or become torn during use, or hands may become contaminated as gloves are removed. Wear a gown, mask, and protective eyewear when the potential exists for any blood or body fluid spattering.

The Public Health Agency of Canada's Routine Practices and Additional Precautions for Preventing the Transmission of Infection in Healthcare Settings (2012) include the most recent epidemiological information for decreasing infection transmission. **Routine practices** (Table 3.2) are intended for use with *all* patients at *all* times regardless of their risk or presumed infection status. They apply to: (a) blood; (b) all body fluids, secretions, and excretions except sweat, regardless of whether they contain visible blood; (c) nonintact skin; and (d) mucous membranes. **Additional precautions** are intended for use when routine practices cannot fully manage the transmissions of the organisms in the health care setting. Routes of transmission have been classified as contact (direct, indirect,

TABLE 3.2   Routine Practice Elements for Use With All Patients

1. Use *point-of-care risk assessment (PCRA)* for each and every patient in the care of your environment. Evaluate the likelihood of exposure, and then chose the appropriate action/personal protective equipment.

2. Perform *hand hygiene* (a) **before** initial patient/patient environmental contact; (b) **before** aseptic procedures; (c) **after** contact with blood, body fluids, secretions, and excretions; (d) **after** contact with any equipment contaminated with body fluids; and (e) **after** removing gloves. Alcohol-based hand rub (ABHR) is the preferred method of hand hygiene in all health care settings.

3. Use *personal protective equipment as required.* Perform hand hygiene prior to donning clean gloves when touching blood, body fluids, secretions, excretions, or items contaminated with these materials; mucous membranes; and nonintact skin. Remove gloves promptly after use, before touching noncontaminated items, and before examining another patient, and wash hands immediately.

   a. *Facial protection: wear a mask, face shield, or mask with visor attachment* that ensures your eyes, nose, mouth, and chin are covered during procedures and during patient care activities that are likely to generate splashes of blood, body fluids, secretions, and excretions or within 2 m of a coughing patient.

   b. *Wear a gown* (clean, nonsterile, appropriate for activity) to protect uncovered skin and clothing during procedures and during patient care activities that are likely to generate splashes of blood, body fluids, secretions, or excretions. Cuffs of gowns should be covered by gloves.

4. *Apply **source control** measures* that identify and contain the source of the pathogen. Triage, respiratory hygiene, patient placement and accommodation, patient flow, handling of deceased bodies, and visitor management all fall under source control.

   a. *Place in a private room* any patient who contaminates the environment or who does not or cannot assist in appropriate hygiene or environmental control. Some transmission-based precautions call for providing single accommodations or other negative-pressure–enhanced environments for certain contact and airborne-transmitted pathogens.

   b. *Be especially careful with used patient care equipment* if it is soiled with blood, body fluids, secretions, and excretions; handle it in a manner that prevents skin and mucous membrane exposure, contamination of clothing, and transfer of microorganisms to other patients and environments. Do not use the reusable equipment on another patient until it has been cleaned and reprocessed appropriately. Discard single-use items appropriately.

Continued

TABLE 3.2   Routine Practice Elements for Use With All Patients—cont'd

c. *Prevent injuries by bloodborne pathogens* when you use or handle needles, scalpels, and other sharp instruments. Never recap used needles, manipulate them with both hands, or direct the point of a needle toward any part of your body; use safety engineered needles at all times when possible as outlined in the *Safer Needles in Healthcare Workplaces Act* of 2006. Do not remove used needles from disposable syringes by hand, and do not otherwise bend, break, or manipulate used needles by hand. Place used disposable syringes, needles, scalpel blades, and other sharp items in appropriate puncture-resistant containers. Use mouthpieces, resuscitation bags, or other ventilation devices instead of mouth-to-mouth resuscitation methods in areas where the need for resuscitation is predictable.

5. Follow *environmental control policies* for the routine care, cleaning, and disinfection of environmental surfaces, beds, bed rails, bedside equipment, and other frequently touched surfaces. Take care with used linen soiled with blood, body fluids, secretions, and excretions; handle, transport, and process this linen in a manner that prevents skin and mucous membrane exposure.

Adapted from Public Health Agency of Canada. (2012). *Routine practices and additional precautions for preventing the transmission of infection in healthcare settings.* Retrieved from http://publications.gc.ca/collections//collection_2013/aspc-phac/HP40-83-2013-eng.pdf.

and droplet), airborne, common vehicle (single contaminated source, such as food), and vector-borne.

THE CLINICAL SETTING

Preparation for a Complete Assessment

Begin by measuring the patient's height, weight, blood pressure, temperature, pulse, and respirations. If needed, measure visual acuity at this time, using the Snellen eye chart.

Ask the patient to change into an examination gown or other clothing that gives you access, leaving his or her underpants on. Unless your assistance is needed, leave the room as the patient undresses.

As you re-enter the room, wash your hands in the patient's presence. Not only is this an infection control measure, but it also demonstrates a readiness to provide safe care.

Explain each step in the examination and how the patient can cooperate. Encourage the patient to ask questions.

Keep your own movements slow, methodical, and deliberate.

As you proceed through the examination, avoid distractions and concentrate on one step at a time. The sequence of the steps may differ, depending on the age of the patient and your own preference. However, you should establish a system that works for you and stick to it to avoid omissions.

Organize the steps so the patient does not change positions too often. Although proper exposure is necessary, use additional drapes to maintain the patient's privacy and to prevent chilling. As you proceed through the examination, ensure that the patient is comfortable with the progression of the assessment.

(See Chapter 20 for the sequence of steps in the complete physical examination.)

Individuals with Acute Health Challenges

For a patient in some distress, alter the position during the examination.

For example, a patient with shortness of breath or ear pain may want to sit up, whereas a patient with faintness or overwhelming fatigue may want to be supine. Initially, it may be necessary just to examine the body areas appropriate to the problem, collecting a **mini-database**. You may resume a complete assessment after the initial distress is resolved.

For more information on the preparation of infants, children, and older adults for the physical examination, see Chapter 9 in Jarvis: *Physical Examination and Health Assessment*, 3rd Canadian edition, pages 149.

CHAPTER 4

General Survey, Measurement, Vital Signs, and Pain Assessment

GENERAL SURVEY

The general survey is a study of the whole person, covering the general health state and any obvious physical characteristics. Objective parameters are used to form the general survey, but these apply to the whole person, not just to one body system.

Begin the general survey at the moment you first encounter the patient. What leaves an immediate impression?

As you proceed through the health history, the measurements, and the vital signs, note the following points that will add up to the general survey: **physical appearance, body structure, mobility,** and **behaviour**.

PHYSICAL APPEARANCE

Age—The person appears his or her stated age.

Sex—Sexual development—Development is appropriate for gender and age.

Level of consciousness—The person is alert and oriented, attends to your questions, and responds appropriately.

Skin colour—Colour tone is even, pigmentation varying with genetic background, and skin is intact with no obvious lesions.

Facial features—Features are symmetrical with movement.

There are no signs of acute distress.

BODY STRUCTURE

Stature—The height appears within normal range for age and genetic heritage.

Nutrition—The weight appears within normal range for height and body build. Body fat distribution is even.

Symmetry—Body parts look equal bilaterally and are in relative proportion to each other.

Posture—The person stands comfortably erect as appropriate for age.

Position—The person sits comfortably in a chair, on the bed, or on the examination table, with arms relaxed at sides and head turned to examiner.

Body build, contour—Normal proportions are:

1. Arm span (fingertip to fingertip) equals height.
2. Body length from crown to pubis is approximately equal to length from pubis to sole.

Obvious physical deformities—Note any congenital or acquired defects.

MOBILITY

Gait—Normally the base width is equal to the shoulder width. Foot placement is accurate. The walk is smooth, even, and well-balanced; associated movements, such as symmetrical arm swing, are present.

Range of motion—Note full mobility for each joint and whether movement is deliberate, accurate, smooth, and coordinated.

No involuntary movement is present.

BEHAVIOUR

Facial expression—The patient maintains eye contact with the examiner (unless a cultural consideration

25

exists). Expressions are appropriate to the situation (e.g., thoughtful, serious, or smiling). Note expressions both while the face is at rest and while the patient is talking.

Mood and affect—The patient is comfortable and cooperative with the examiner and interacts pleasantly.

Speech—Articulation (the ability to form words) is clear and understandable. The stream of speech is fluent, with an even pace. Ideas are conveyed clearly. Word choice is appropriate to culture and education.

The patient communicates in his or her native language easily by himself or herself or with an interpreter.

Dress—Clothing is appropriate for the climate, looks clean, and fits the body, and is appropriate for the patient's culture and age group.

Personal hygiene—The patient appears clean and groomed appropriately for his or her age, occupation, and socioeconomic group. Hair is groomed or brushed. Makeup is appropriate for age and culture.

MEASUREMENT

WEIGHT

Use a standardized balance or electronic standing scale. Instruct the patient to remove his or her shoes and heavy outer clothing before standing on the scale. When a sequence of repeated weights is necessary, aim for approximately the same time of day and the same type of clothing worn each time. Record the weight in kilograms and in pounds. Show the patient how his or her own weight compares with the recommended range for height.

Compare the patient's weight with that from the previous health visit. A recent weight loss may be explained by successful dieting.

An unexplained weight loss may be a sign of a short-term illness (e.g., fever, infection, disease of the mouth or throat) or a chronic illness (endocrine disease, malignancy, mental health illness).

A weight gain usually reflects overabundant caloric intake, unhealthy eating habits, a sedentary lifestyle, or fluid accumulation. Unexplained weight gain may indicate fluid retention (e.g. heart failure) (McGee, 2018).

HEIGHT

Use a wall-mounted device or the measuring pole on the balance scale. Align the extended headpiece with the top of the head. The patient should be shoeless, standing straight with gentle traction under the jaw, and looking straight ahead. Feet, shoulders, and buttocks should be in contact with a hard surface.

BODY MASS INDEX

Body mass index (BMI) is a practical marker of optimal weight for height and an indicator of obesity or protein-calorie malnutrition. BMI is calculated as follows:

$$BMI = \frac{Weight\ (in\ kilograms)}{Height\ (in\ metres)^2}$$

or

$$\frac{Weight\ (in\ pounds)}{Height\ (in\ inches)^2} \times 703$$

For a quick determination of BMI, use a straight edge to help locate the point on the chart where height (centimetres or inches) and weight (kilograms or

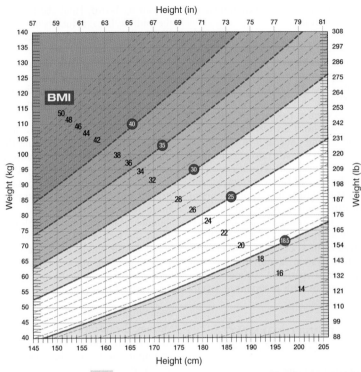

4.1 Body mass index (BMI) nomogram.

pounds) intersect (Fig. 4.1). Read the number on the dashed line closest to this point.

The following BMI interpretations are used for adults (World Health Organization [WHO], 2017):

<18.5	Underweight
18.5 to 24.9	Normal weight
25.0 to 29.9	Overweight
30.0 to 34.9	Obesity (Class 1)
35 to 39.9	Obesity (Class 2)
≥40	Extreme obesity (Class 3)

Children 2 to 19 years of age who are in the 97th to 99th percentile or beyond require further assessment and intervention (Canadian Paediatric Society, 2014).

WAIST-TO-HIP RATIO

The waist-to-hip ratio reflects body fat distribution as an indicator of health risk. Patients with obesity who have a greater proportion of fat in the upper body, especially in the abdomen, have android obesity; obese patients with most of their fat in the hips and thighs have gynoid obesity. The equation is as follows:

$$\text{Waist-to-hip ratio} = \frac{\text{Waist circumference}}{\text{Hip circumference}}$$

where waist circumference is measured at the smallest circumference below the rib cage and above the iliac crest, and hip circumference is measured at the largest circumference of the buttocks.

In addition, **waist circumference** alone can be used to predict greater health risk. Measure at the end of gentle expiration. A waist circumference higher than 88 cm (35 in) in women and higher than 102 cm (40 in) in men places them at risk for type 2 diabetes, coronary heart disease, and hypertension (Health Canada, 2016).

Health Canada (2016) guidelines for body weight classification in adults use BMI measurement and waist circumference as indicators of health risk. It is important to recognize that weight classification is only a component of a comprehensive health assessment. This classification system is not intended for use with patients younger than 18 years or with pregnant or lactating women.

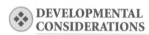

DEVELOPMENTAL CONSIDERATIONS

Infants and Children

Weight

Weigh an infant on a platform-type balance scale. To check calibration, set the weight at zero and observe the beam balance. Guard the baby so that he or she does not fall. Weigh to the nearest 10 g (1/2 oz) for infants and 100 g (1/4 lb) for toddlers.

For children 2 or 3 years of age, use the upright scale. Leave underpants on the child. Some young children are fearful of the rickety standing platform and may prefer sitting on the infant scale. Use the upright scale with preschool- and school-age children, maintaining modesty with light clothing.

Length

For a child younger than 2 years, measure the body length when the child is supine by using a horizontal measuring board. Hold the head in the midline. Because infants normally flex their legs, extend the legs momentarily by holding the knees together and pushing them down until the legs are flat on the table. Avoid using a tape measure along the infant's length because this method yields inaccurate results.

For a child 2 or 3 years of age, measure the height by standing the child against the pole on the platform scale or against a flat ruler taped to the wall. Encourage the child to stand straight and tall and to look straight ahead without tilting the head. The shoulders, buttocks, and heels should touch the wall. Hold a book or flat board on the child's head at a right angle to the wall. Mark just under the book or board, noting the measure to the nearest 1 mm (1/8 in).

Head Circumference

Measure the infant's head circumference at birth and at each well-child visit up to age 2 years, then yearly up to 6 years. Circle the tape around the head at the prominent frontal and occipital bones; the widest span is correct. Plot the measurement on standardized growth charts. Compare the infant's head size with that expected for age. A series of measurements is more valuable than a single figure to show the *rate* of head growth.

The newborn's head measures about 32 to 38 cm (average about 34 cm) and is about 2 cm larger than the chest circumference. The chest grows at a faster rate than the cranium; at some time between 6 months and 2 years, both measurements are about the same, and after 2 years, the chest circumference is greater than the head circumference.

Measurement of the chest circumference is valuable in a comparison with the head circumference, but not necessarily by itself. Encircle the tape around the chest at the nipple line. It should be snug, but not so tight that it leaves a mark.

Older Adults

Weight

Older adults appear sharper in contour with more prominent bony landmarks than are found in younger adults. Body weight decreases during the 80s and 90s. This factor is more evident in males, perhaps because of greater muscle shrinkage. The distribution of fat also changes during the 80s and 90s. Even with good nutrition, subcutaneous fat is lost from the face and periphery (especially the forearms), whereas additional fat is deposited on the abdomen and hips.

Height

By the 80s and 90s, many people are shorter than they were in their 70s. This results from shortening in the spinal column, which is caused by thinning of the vertebral discs and shortening of the individual vertebrae, as well as slight flexion in the knees and hips and the postural changes of kyphosis. Because long bones do not shorten with age, the overall body proportion looks different; a shorter trunk with relatively long extremities.

VITAL SIGNS

TEMPERATURE

The normal oral temperature in a resting patient ranges from 35.8 to 37.3°C (96.4 to 99.1°F) (mean, 37°C [98.6°F]). The rectal temperature measures 0.4°C to 0.5°C (0.7° to 1°F) higher. The normal temperature is influenced by:

- A diurnal cycle of 1°C to 1.5°C; the trough occurs in the early morning hours, and the peak occurs in late afternoon to early evening.
- The menstruation cycle in women. Progesterone secretion, occurring with ovulation at midcycle, causes a 0.5°C to 1.0°C rise in temperature that continues until menses.
- Exercise. Moderate to strenuous exercise increases body temperature.
- Age. Wider normal variations occur in infants and young children as a result of less effective heat control mechanisms. In older adults, temperature is usually lower than in other age groups with a mean of 36.2°C (97.2°F).

The **axillary temperature** is safe and accurate for infants and young children when the environment can be controlled. It is not the method of choice in adults as it is highly insensitive.

The **electronic thermometer** has the advantages of providing swift and accurate measurements (usually in 20 to 30 seconds) as well as safe, unbreakable, disposable probe covers. The instrument must be fully charged and correctly calibrated.

Shake a mercury-free **glass thermometer** down to a reading of around 35.5°C (96°F), and place the thermometer at the base of the tongue in either of the posterior sublingual pockets, *not* in front of the tongue. Instruct the patient to keep his or her lips closed. Leave the thermometer in place 3 to 4 minutes if the patient is afebrile and up to 8 minutes if the patient is febrile. Wait 20 minutes before taking the temperature if the person has just taken hot or iced liquids and 2 minutes if he or she has just smoked.

The **tympanic membrane thermometer** (TMT) is a noninvasive, nontraumatic device that is extremely quick and efficient. The probe tip has the shape of an otoscope, the

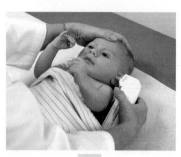

4.2

instrument used to inspect the ear. Cover the probe tip with a tip cover, and gently place the probe tip in the patient's ear canal. Do not force it in, and do not occlude the canal. Activate the device, and you can read the temperature in 2 to 3 seconds (Fig. 4.2).

The newest noninvasive temperature measurement method uses infrared emissions from the temporal artery. The **temporal artery thermometer** (TAT) is used by sliding the probe across the forehead and behind the ear. The thermometer works by taking multiple readings and providing an average. The reading takes approximately 6 seconds. This approach is well tolerated and is more accurate than TMTs; however, there are conflicting reports about its accuracy (Holzhauer et al., 2009).

Measure the **rectal temperature** only when the other routes are not practical—for example, in comatose or confused patients, those in shock, or those who cannot close the mouth because of breathing or oxygen tubes, wired mandible, or other facial dysfunction—or if no tympanic membrane thermometer equipment is available. Wear gloves, insert a lubricated rectal probe cover on an electric thermometer, and insert the thermometer only 2 to 3 cm (1 in) into the adult rectum, directed toward the umbilicus. (For a glass thermometer, leave in place for 2.5 minutes.)

PULSE

Using the pads of your first three fingers, palpate the radial pulse at the flexor aspect of the wrist laterally along the radius bone. Press until you feel the strongest pulsation. If the rhythm is regular, count the number of beats in 30 seconds and multiply by 2. If, however, the rhythm is irregular, count for 1 full minute.

In the adult at physical and mental rest, recent clinical evidence shows the normal resting heart range of 95% of healthy persons at 50 to 95 beats per minute (bpm). Well-trained athletes normally have a resting rate as low as 50 bpm. The rate varies with gender; after puberty, girls have a slightly faster rate.

RESPIRATIONS

Normally, a patient's breathing is relaxed, regular, automatic, and silent. Because most people are unaware of their breathing, do not mention that you will be counting the respirations; the patient's awareness that you are doing so may alter the normal pattern. Instead, maintain your position of counting the radial pulse, and unobtrusively count the respirations. Count for 30 seconds if respirations are normal or for 1 full minute if you suspect an abnormality. Avoid the 15-second interval because the result can vary by a factor of ± 4, which is significant with such a small number.

Respiratory rates are 10 to 20 breaths per minute for adults and are normally more rapid for infants and children. A fairly constant ratio of pulse rate to respiratory rate also exists, which is about 4:1. Normally, both pulse and respiratory rates rise as a response to exercise or anxiety.

BLOOD PRESSURE

Blood pressure (BP) is the force of the blood pushing against the side of the vessel wall. The **systolic**

pressure is the maximum pressure felt on the artery during left ventricular contraction, or systole. The **diastolic pressure** is the elastic recoil, or resting, pressure that the blood exerts constantly between each contraction. The **pulse pressure** is the difference between the systolic and diastolic pressures and reflects the stroke volume.

The average BP in young adults is influenced by a variety of factors, such as:

Age: Normally BP rises gradually through childhood and into adult years.

Sex: Before puberty, there is no difference between males and females. After puberty, females usually have a lower BP than do male counterparts. After menopause, BP is higher in women than in male counterparts.

Ethnocultural considerations: In Canada, adults of African descent usually have a higher BP than do those of European descent of the same age. The incidence of hypertension is twice as high among those of African descent; reasons for the difference are not fully understood, but it appears to be a result of genetic and environmental factors.

Diurnal rhythm: A daily cycle of a peak and a trough occurs: The BP is highest in late afternoon or early evening and then declines to an early morning low.

Weight: BP is higher in obese persons than in persons of normal weight of the same age (including adolescents).

Exercise: Increasing activity yields a proportionate increase in BP. Within 5 minutes of terminating the exercise, the BP normally returns to baseline.

Emotions: The BP momentarily rises with fear, anger, and pain as a result of stimulation of the sympathetic nervous system.

Stress: The BP is elevated in patients feeling continual tension because of lifestyle, occupational stress, or life problems.

BP is measured with a stethoscope and an aneroid *sphygmomanometer.*

The cuff consists of an inflatable rubber bladder inside a cloth cover. The width of the rubber bladder should equal 40% of the circumference of the patient's arm. The length of the bladder should equal 80% of this circumference.

The cuff size is important; using a cuff that is too narrow yields a falsely high BP because it takes extra pressure to compress the artery. Match the appropriate size cuff to the patient's arm size and shape and not to the patient's age.

The Procedure: Arm Pressure

A comfortable, relaxed patient yields a valid BP. Many patients are anxious at the beginning of an examination; allow at least a 5-minute rest before measuring the BP.

Take three BP measurements separated by 2 minutes; discard the first reading; and average the other two. This procedure is the new recommended Canadian standard (Canadian Hypertension Education Program [CHEP], 2016).

The patient may be sitting or lying, with the bare arm supported at the heart level. Palpate the brachial artery, which is located just above the antecubital fossa, medial to the biceps tendon. With the cuff deflated, centre it about 2.5 cm (1 in) above the brachial artery, and wrap it evenly around the arm.

Now palpate the brachial or radial artery. Inflate the cuff until the artery pulsation is obliterated and then 20 to 30 mm Hg beyond. This will avoid missing an **auscultatory gap,** which is a period when Korotkoff's sounds disappear during auscultation. This is common with hypertension.

Deflate the cuff quickly and completely, then wait 15 to 30 seconds before reinflating so that the blood trapped in the veins can dissipate.

Place the bell of the stethoscope over the site of the brachial artery, making a light but airtight seal. Use the bell endpiece if you have one (Fig. 4.3). Rapidly inflate the cuff to the maximal inflation level that you determined. Then deflate the cuff slowly and evenly, about 2 mm Hg per heartbeat. Note the points at which you hear the first appearance of sound, the muffling of sound, and the final disappearance of sound. These are phases I, IV, and V of **Korotkoff's sounds**.

For all age groups, the fifth Korotkoff phase is now used to define diastolic pressure. When a variance

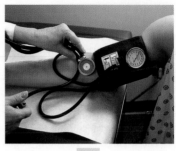

4.3

greater than 10 to 12 mm Hg exists between phases IV and V, however, record *both* phases along with the systolic reading (e.g., 142/98/80). Table 4.1 presents a list of common errors in BP measurement.

TABLE 4.1	Common Errors in Blood Pressure Measurement	
Common Error	Result	Rationale
Taking blood pressure reading when patient is anxious or angry or has just been active	Falsely high	Sympathetic nervous system stimulation
Faulty arm position		
Above level of heart	Falsely low	Eliminates effect of hydrostatic pressure
Below level of heart	Falsely high	Additional force of gravity added to brachial artery pressure
Patient supports own arm	Falsely high diastolic	Sustained isometric muscular contraction
Faulty leg position (e.g., patient's legs are crossed)	Falsely high systolic and diastolic	Translocation of blood volume from dependent legs to thoracic area
Examiner's eyes are not level with meniscus of mercury column		
Looking up at meniscus	Falsely high	Parallax
Looking down on meniscus	Falsely low	
Inaccurate cuff size (the most common error)		
Cuff too narrow for extremity	Falsely high	Excessive pressure needed to occlude brachial artery
Cuff wrap is too loose or uneven, or bladder balloons out of wrap	Falsely high	Excessive pressure needed to occlude brachial artery

TABLE 4.1	Common Errors in Blood Pressure Measurement—cont'd	
Common Error	Result	Rationale
Failure to palpate radial artery while cuff is inflated	Falsely low systolic	Missing initial systolic tapping or tuning in during *auscultatory gap* (tapping sounds disappear for 10–40 mm Hg and then return; common with hypertension)
Poor inflation of the cuff		
Overinflation of the cuff	Pain	
Pushing stethoscope too hard on brachial artery	Falsely low diastolic	Distortion of artery by excessive pressure so that the sounds continue
Deflating cuff:		
Too quickly	Falsely low systolic or falsely high diastolic	Insufficient time to hear tapping
Too slowly	Falsely high diastolic	Venous congestion in forearm makes sounds less audible
Halting during descent and reinflating cuff to recheck systolic	Falsely high diastolic	Venous congestion in forearm
Failure to wait 1–2 min before repeating entire reading	Falsely high diastolic	Venous congestion in forearm
Any observer error	Any error	
Examiner's haste		
Faulty technique		
Examiner's digit preference, "hears" more results that end in zero than would occur by chance alone (e.g., 130/80)		
Diminished hearing acuity		
Defective or inaccurately calibrated equipment		

Take serial measurements of pulse and BP when you suspect volume depletion; when the patient is known to have hypertension or is taking antihypertensive medications; or when the patient reports fainting or syncope. Have the patient rest supine for 2 or 3 minutes, take baseline readings of pulse and BP, and then repeat the measurements with the patient sitting and then standing. A slight decrease (less than 10 mm Hg) in systolic pressure is normal when the position is changed from supine to standing.

Orthostatic hypotension—a drop in systolic pressure of more than 20 mm Hg, or an orthostatic pulse increase of 20 bpm or more—occurs with a quick change to a standing position. It is due to abrupt peripheral vasodilation without a compensatory increase in cardiac output. Orthostatic changes also occur with prolonged bed rest, older age, hypovolemia, and ingestion of some medications. Figure 4.4 presents

Notes:

1. If AOBP is used, use the mean calculated and displayed by the device. If non-AOBP (see note 2) is used, take at least three readings, discard the first and calculate the mean of the remaining measurements. A history and physical exam should be performed and diagnostic tests ordered.

2. **AOBP** = Automated Office BP. This is performed with the patient unattended in a private area. **Non-AOBP** = Non-automated measurement performed using an electronic upper arm device with the provider in the room.

3. Diagnostic thresholds for AOBP, ABPM, and home BP in patients with diabetes have yet to be established (and may be lower than 130/80 mmHg).

4. Serial office measurements over 3–5 visits can be used if ABPM or home measurement not available.

5. Home BP Series: Two readings taken each morning and evening for 7 days (28 total). Discard first day readings and average the last 6 days.

6. Annual BP measurement is recommended to detect progression to hypertension.

Elevated BP Reading (office, home, or pharmacy)

Dedicated Office Visit[1] Mean Office BP ≥ 180/110

— YES → **Hypertension**

— NO →

No Diabetes	Diabetes[3]
1. AOBP[2] ≥135/85 (preferred)	AOBP or non-AOBP[2] ≥130/80
OR	
2. Non-AOBP[2] ≥140/90 (if AOBP unavailable)	

— NO → **No Hypertension[6]**

— YES →

Out-of-office Measurement[4]
1. ABPM (preferred) Daytime mean ≥135/85 24-hour mean ≥130/80
OR
2. Home BP Series[5] Mean ≥135/85

— YES → **Hypertension**

— NO → **White Coat Hypertension[6]**

4.4 Hypertension diagnostic algorithm. *ABPM,* Ambulatory blood pressure measurement; *AOBP,* automated office blood pressure; *BP,* blood pressure.

further information on Canadian recommendations for the assessment of hypertensive patients.

✦ DEVELOPMENTAL CONSIDERATIONS

The aorta and major arteries tend to harden with age. As the heart pumps against a stiffer aorta, the systolic pressure increases, causing pulse pressure to increase. With many older people, both the systolic and diastolic pressures increase, making it difficult to distinguish normal aging values from abnormal hypertension.

THE DOPPLER TECHNIQUE

The Doppler technique is used to locate the peripheral pulse sites. For BP measurement, the Doppler technique augments Korotkoff sounds when they are hard to hear with a stethoscope, such as in critically ill individuals with a low BP, in infants with small arms, and in obese patients in whom the sounds are muffled by layers of fat. Proper cuff placement is also difficult on an obese patient's cone-shaped upper arm. In this situation, you can place the cuff on the more even forearm and hold the Doppler probe over the radial artery (Fig. 4.5). For either location, use the following procedure:
- Apply coupling gel to the transducer probe.
- Turn the Doppler flowmeter on.

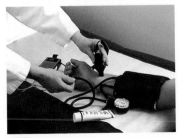

4.5 Measuring blood pressure using the Doppler technique.

- Touch the probe to the skin, holding the probe perpendicular to the artery.
- A pulsatile whooshing sound indicates location of the artery. You may need to rotate the probe, but maintain contact with the skin. Do not push the probe too hard or you will obliterate the pulse.
- Inflate the cuff until the sounds disappear, then inflate another 20 to 30 mm Hg beyond that point.
- Slowly deflate the cuff, noting the point at which the first whooshing sounds appear. This is the systolic pressure.
- It is difficult to hear the muffling of sound or a reliable disappearance of sounds indicating the diastolic pressure (phases IV and V of Korotkoff sounds). However, the systolic blood pressure alone is valuable data about the level of tissue perfusion and about blood flow through patent vessels.

PAIN ASSESSMENT

Pain is a highly complex and subjective experience that originates from the central nervous system (CNS), the peripheral nervous system, or both. "Pain is whatever the experiencing person says it is, existing whenever he says it does" (McCaffery, 1968, page 95). Since pain is a subjective experience, the self-report of pain is the most reliable indicator that an individual is experiencing pain. With knowledge that pain occurs on a neurochemical level, the clinician cannot base the diagnosis of pain exclusively on physical exam findings. Physical exam findings can lend support.

Pain is multidimensional in scope, encompassing physical, affective, and functional domains. Various tools have been developed to capture unidimensional aspects (e.g., intensity) or multidimensional components (e.g., effect on activities of daily living and quality of life). Select the pain

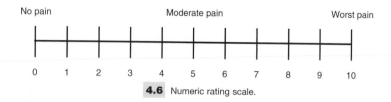

No pain   Moderate pain   Worst pain

0   1   2   3   4   5   6   7   8   9   10

4.6 Numeric rating scale.

assessment tool based on its purpose, time involved in administration, and the patient's ability to comprehend and complete the tool.

Pain rating scales are unidimensional and are intended to reflect pain intensity. They come in various forms. Pain rating scales can be used to ascertain baseline intensity, track changes, and give some degree of evaluation to a treatment modality. **Numeric rating scales** ask the patient to choose a number that rates the level of pain, wherein 0 represents no pain and 10 indicates the worst possible pain. It can be administered verbally or visually along a vertical or horizontal line (Fig. 4.6).

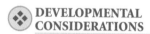 **DEVELOPMENTAL CONSIDERATIONS**

Infants

Infants have the same capacity for pain as do adults. Preverbal infants are at higher risk for undertreatment of pain because of the persistent belief that infants do not remember pain. Because neonates and young infants are preverbal and incapable of self-report, pain assessment is dependent upon behavioural and physiological clues.

Toddlers and children older than 2 years of age can report pain and point to its location. They cannot rate pain intensity at this developmental level. It is helpful to ask the parent or caregiver what words their child uses

to report pain (e.g., "boo-boo," "owie"). Be aware that some children will try to act "grown up and brave" and often deny having pain in the presence of a stranger, or if they are fearful of receiving a "shot."

Rating scales can be administered to patients aged 4 or 5 years. The Faces Pain Scale—Revised (FPS-R) tool has six drawings of faces that show pain intensity, from "no pain" on the left (score of 0) to "very much pain" on the right (score of 10). The child is asked to select the face that best represents his or her pain intensity. Numbers are not shown to children, but the number scoring makes this tool compatible with the widely used 0-to-10 metric for numeric pain scales. (See Chapter 11 in Jarvis: *Physical Examination & Health Assessment*, 3rd Canadian edition, pages 190.)

Older Adults

No evidence exists to suggest that older individuals perceive pain to a lesser degree or that sensitivity is diminished with age. Although pain is a common experience among older individuals, it is *not* a normal process of aging. Pain indicates disease or injury.

Older adults may find the numerical scale too abstract and may respond to scales in which words are used. An alternative is the simple **Descriptor Scale,** which lists words that describe different levels of pain intensity, such as *no pain, mild pain, moderate pain,* and *severe pain.*

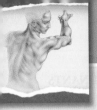

CHAPTER 5

Skin, Hair, and Nails

STRUCTURE AND FUNCTION

The skin has two layers: the outer highly differentiated *epidermis* and the inner supportive *dermis* (Fig. 5.1). Beneath these layers is a third layer, the insulating *subcutaneous* layer of adipose tissue.

The **sebaceous** glands produce a protective lipid, *sebum*, which is secreted through the hair follicles. The **eccrine** glands are coiled tubules that open directly onto the skin surface and produce a dilute saline solution called *sweat*, which helps reduce body temperature. The **apocrine** glands open into hair follicles, become active during puberty, and produce a thick, milky secretion with emotional and sexual stimulation.

The nails are hard plates of keratin on the dorsal edges of the fingers and toes (Fig. 5.2). The nail plate is clear, with fine longitudinal ridges that become prominent in aging. Nails take their pink colour from the underlying nail bed of highly vascular epithelial cells.

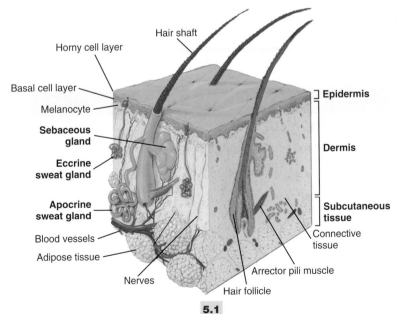

5.1

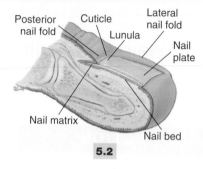

Posterior nail fold
Cuticle
Lunula
Lateral nail fold
Nail plate
Nail matrix
Nail bed

5.2

SOCIAL DETERMINANTS OF HEALTH CONSIDERATIONS

Melanin is responsible for the various colours and tones of skin among people from culturally diverse backgrounds. Melanin protects the skin against harmful ultraviolet rays, a genetic advantage accounting for the lower incidence of skin cancer among individuals of African, Indian, or Indigenous descent with dark skin.

SUBJECTIVE DATA

1. Previous history of skin disease (allergies, hives, psoriasis, eczema)
2. Change in pigmentation
3. Change in mole (size or colour)
4. Excessive dryness or moisture
5. Pruritus
6. Excessive bruising
7. Rash or lesion
8. Medications (any that cause allergic skin response, increased sunlight sensitivity)
9. Hair loss
10. Change in nails
11. Environmental or occupational hazards (sun exposure, toxic chemicals, insect bites)
12. Self-care behaviours (daily hygiene; use of soaps, cosmetics, or chemicals)

OBJECTIVE DATA

EQUIPMENT NEEDED

Strong direct lighting (natural daylight is ideal to evaluate skin characteristics; halogen light will suffice)
Small centimetre ruler
Penlight
Gloves

Normal Range of Findings	Abnormal Findings

Inspect and Palpate the Skin

Colour

General Pigmentation. The skin tone is consistent with genetic background and varies from pinkish tan to ruddy dark tan or from light to dark brown and may have yellow or olive overtones. Dark-skinned people normally have areas of lighter pigmentation on the palms, nail beds, and lips.

General pigmentation is darker in sun-exposed areas. Common (benign) pigmentations also occur:

- **Freckles** (ephelides): small, flat macules of brown melanin pigment that occur on sun-exposed skin.
- **Mole** (nevus): a proliferation of melanocytes, tan to brown colour, flat or raised; characterized by their symmetry, small size (6 mm or less), smooth borders, and single uniform pigmentation.
- **Birthmarks:** may be tan to brown colour.

Advise anyone with moles or birthmarks to perform periodic skin self-examinations. Watch for danger signs listed here. Ask a family member to check any areas the patient cannot see (e.g., the back).

Danger signs: Abnormal characteristics of pigmented lesions are summarized with the mnemonic **ABCDE:**

Asymmetry (*not* regularly round or oval, two halves of lesion do not look the same)

Border irregularity (notching, scalloping, ragged edges or poorly defined margins)

Colour variation (areas of brown, tan, black, blue, red, white, or combination)

Diameter greater than 6 mm (i.e., the size of a pencil eraser), although early melanomas may be diagnosed at a smaller size

Elevation and **E**volution

Additionally, an individual may report a rapidly changing lesion, a new pigmented lesion, or the development of itching, burning, or bleeding in a mole. Any of these signs should raise suspicion of malignant melanoma and warrant referral.

Continued

Normal Range of Findings	Abnormal Findings

Widespread Colour Change. Note any colour change in skin over the entire body, such as pallor (white), erythema (red), cyanosis (blue), and jaundice (yellow). In dark-skinned people, the amount of normal pigment may mask colour changes. Lips and nail beds show some colour change, but they vary with the person's skin colour and may not always be accurate signs. The more reliable sites are those with the least pigmentation, such as under the tongue, the buccal mucosa, the palpebral conjunctiva, and the sclera. Table 5.1 lists specific clues to assessment.

Temperature

Use the backs (dorsa) of your hands and palpate bilaterally. The skin should be warm with equal temperature bilaterally. Hands and feet may be slightly cooler in a cool environment.

Hypothermia. Generalized coolness may be induced, such as in hypothermia used for surgery or high fever. Localized coolness is expected with an immobilized extremity, as when a limb is in a cast, or with an intravenous infusion.

General hypothermia accompanies central circulatory problems such as shock. Localized hypothermia occurs in peripheral arterial insufficiency and Raynaud's disease.

Hyperthermia. Generalized hyperthermia occurs with an increased metabolic rate, such as in fever or after heavy exercise. A localized area feels hyperthermic with trauma, infection, or sunburn.

Hyperthyroidism produces an increase in metabolic rate, causing warmth and moistness of skin.

Moisture

Perspiration appears normally on the face, hands, axilla, and skinfolds in response to activity, a warm environment, or anxiety. **Diaphoresis,** or profuse perspiration, accompanies an increase in metabolic rate, as occurs in strenuous activity or fever.

Diaphoresis occurs with thyrotoxicosis and with stimulation of the nervous system with anxiety or pain.

Look for **dehydration** in the oral mucous membranes. Normally, there is none, and the mucous membranes look smooth and moist. Be aware that dark skin may normally look dry and flaky, but this does not necessarily indicate systemic dehydration.

With dehydration, mucous membranes look dry and the lips look parched and cracked. With extreme dryness, the skin is fissured, resembling cracks in a dry lake bed.

Normal Range of Findings	Abnormal Findings

Texture

Normal skin feels smooth and firm, with an even surface.

Hyperthyroidism: skin feels smoother and softer, like velvet.

Hypothyroidism: skin feels rough, dry, and flaky.

Thickness

The epidermis is uniformly thin over most of the body, although thickened callus areas are normal on palms and soles. A callus is a circumscribed overgrowth of epidermis and is an adaptation to excessive pressure from the friction of work and weight bearing.

Skin is very thin and shiny (atrophic) with arterial insufficiency.

Edema

Edema is fluid accumulating in the intercellular spaces and is not normally present. To check for edema, imprint your thumbs firmly against the ankle malleolus or the tibia. Normally, the skin surface resumes its smoothness immediately. If your pressure leaves a dent in the skin, "pitting" edema is present. Its presence is graded on a four-point scale:

1+: Mild pitting, slight indentation, no perceptible swelling of the leg
2+: Moderate pitting, indentation subsides rapidly
3+: Deep pitting, indentation remains for a short time, leg looks swollen
4+: Very deep pitting, indentation lasts a long time, leg is very swollen and distorted

This scale is somewhat subjective; ratings vary among examiners.

Edema masks normal skin colour and obscures pathological conditions such as jaundice or cyanosis because the fluid lies between the surface and the pigmented and vascular layers. It makes dark skin look lighter.

Edema is most evident in dependent parts of the body (feet, ankles, and sacral areas), where the skin looks puffy and tight. Edema makes the hair follicles more prominent, so you note a pigskin or orange-peel look (*peau d'orange*).

Unilateral edema: consider a local or peripheral cause.

Bilateral edema or edema that is generalized over the whole body (*anasarca*) suggests a central problem, such as heart failure or kidney failure.

Continued

Normal Range of Findings	Abnormal Findings

Mobility and Turgor

Pinch up a large fold of skin on the anterior chest under the clavicle. Mobility is the skin's ease of rising, and turgor is its ability to return to place promptly when released. Together, they reflect the elasticity of the skin.

Mobility is decreased when edema is present.

Poor turgor is evident in severe dehydration or extreme weight loss; the pinched skin recedes slowly or "tents" and stands by itself.

Vascularity or Bruising

Cherry (senile) angiomas are small (1–5 mm), smooth, slightly raised, bright red dots that commonly appear on the trunk in all adults older than 30 years. They normally increase in size and number with aging and are not significant.

Any bruising (ecchymosis) should be consistent with the expected trauma of life. There are normally no venous dilations or varicosities.

Multiple bruises at different stages of healing and excessive bruises above the knees or elbows should raise concern about physical abuse.

Needle marks or tracks from intravenous injection of street drugs may be visible on the antecubital fossae, on the forearms, or over any available vein.

Document the presence of any tattoos (a permanent skin design from indelible pigment) on the person's chart. Advise the patient that the use of tattoo needles and tattoo parlour equipment of doubtful sterility increases the risk of hepatitis C.

Lesions

If any lesions are present, note these characteristics:
1. Colour.
2. Elevation: flat, raised, or pedunculated.
3. Pattern or shape: the grouping or distinctness of each lesion; for example, annular, grouped, confluent, or linear. The pattern may be characteristic of a certain disease.
4. Size, in centimetres: use a ruler to measure. Avoid descriptions such as "quarter size" or "pea size."
5. Location and distribution on body: is it generalized or localized to area of a specific irritant (around jewellery, a watchband, eyes)?
6. Any exudate: colour and any odour.

Lesions are traumatic or pathological changes in previously normal structures. When a lesion develops on previously unaltered skin, it is **primary.** When a lesion changes over time or changes because of a factor such as scratching or infection, it is **secondary.**

Normal Range of Findings	Abnormal Findings
Wear a glove if you anticipate contact with mucosa, blood, any other body fluid, or an open skin lesion.	See Table 5.2 for the patterns and Tables 5.3 and 5.4 for the characteristics of primary and secondary skin lesions.

Inspect and Palpate the Hair

Colour

Hair colour comes from melanin production and may vary from pale blond to totally black. Greying normally begins as early as the third decade of life because of reduced melanin production in the follicles.

Texture

Scalp hair may be fine or thick and may look straight, curly, or kinky. It should look shiny, although this characteristic may be lost with the use of some beauty products such as dyes, rinses, or perm materials.

Note dull, coarse, or brittle scalp hair.

Lesions

All areas of the scalp should be clean and free of any lesions or pest inhabitants. Many people normally have seborrhea (dandruff), which is characterized by loose white flakes.

Distinguish dandruff from nits (eggs) of lice, which are oval, adhere to the hair shaft, and cause intense itching.

Inspect and Palpate the Nails

Shape and Contour

The nail surface is normally slightly curved or flat, and the posterior and lateral nail folds are smooth and rounded. Nail edges are smooth, rounded, and clean, suggesting adequate self-care.

Chronic iron-deficiency anemia may present with "spoon" nails, a concave shape.

Paronychia (red, swollen, tender inflammation of the nail folds) occurs with trauma or infection.

Jagged nails, nails bitten to the quick, or traumatized nail folds from chronic nervous picking suggest nervous habits.

Chronically dirty nails suggest poor self-care or chronic staining of some occupations.

Continued

Normal Range of Findings	Abnormal Findings
The Profile Sign. View the index finger at its profile and note the angle of the nail base; it should be about 160 degrees. The nail base is firm to palpation. Curved nails with a convex profile are a variation of normal. They may look like clubbed nails, but the angle between nail base and nail is normal (i.e., 160 degrees or less).	Clubbing of nails occurs with congenital, chronic, and cyanotic heart disease and with emphysema and chronic bronchitis. In early clubbing, the angle straightens out to 180 degrees, and the nail base feels spongy to palpation. (see Fig. 13.9, page 239 in Jarvis: *Physical Examination and Health Assessment,* 3rd Canadian edition.)
Consistency	
The nail surface is smooth and regular, not brittle or splitting.	Pits, transverse grooves, or lines may indicate a nutrient deficiency or may accompany acute illness in which nail growth is disturbed.
Nail thickness is uniform.	Nails are thickened and ridged with arterial insufficiency.
The nail is firmly adherent to the nail bed, and the nail base is firm to palpation.	A spongy nail base accompanies clubbing.
Colour	
The translucent nail plate shows an even, pink nail bed underneath.	Cyanosis or marked pallor.
Dark-skinned people may have brown-black pigmented areas or linear bands or streaks along the nail edge. All people normally may have white hairline linear markings (leukonychia striata) from trauma or picking at the cuticle. Note any abnormal markings in the nail beds.	Brown linear streaks (especially sudden appearance) are abnormal in light-skinned people and may indicate melanoma.
Capillary Refill. Depress the nail edge to cause blanching, and then release, noting the return of colour. Normally, colour returns instantly or at least within a few seconds in a cold environment. This indicates the status of the peripheral circulation. A sluggish colour return takes longer than 1 or 2 seconds.	Splinter hemorrhages occur with subacute bacterial endocarditis; transverse ridges, or Beau's lines, occur with trauma.
	Cyanotic nail beds or sluggish colour return may be indicative of cardiovascular or respiratory dysfunction.

Normal Range of Findings	Abnormal Findings

DEVELOPMENTAL CONSIDERATIONS

Infants

Skin Colour: General Pigmentation. Newborns of African descent initially have lighter toned skin than their parents. Their full melanotic colour is evident in the nail beds and scrotal folds. The **Mongolian spot** is a common variation of hyperpigmentation in newborns of Indigenous, African, East Indian, or Hispanic descent as a result of deep dermal melanocytes. It is a blue-black to purple macular area at the sacrum or buttocks, but sometimes it occurs on the abdomen, thighs, shoulders, or arms. It gradually fades during the first year.

Bruising is a common soft tissue injury that follows a rapid, traumatic, or breech birth.

Multiple bruises in various stages of healing, or pattern injury, suggest child abuse.

Adolescents

The increase in sebaceous gland activity creates increased oiliness and **acne**. Acne lesions usually appear on the face and sometimes on the chest, back, and shoulders.

Pregnant Women

Striae are jagged linear "stretch marks" coloured silver to pink that appear during the second trimester on the abdomen, breasts, and sometimes on the thighs. They occur in one half of all pregnancies and fade after delivery, but do not disappear. On the abdomen, the **linea nigra** appears as a brownish black line down the midline.

Chloasma is an irregular brown patch of hyperpigmentation on the face. It may occur with pregnancy or in women taking oral contraceptive pills. Chloasma disappears after delivery or after the woman stops taking the pills.

Vascular spiders occur in two-thirds of all pregnancies, primarily in Canadians of European descent. These lesions have tiny red centres with radiating branches and occur on the face, neck, upper chest, and arms.

Continued

Normal Range of Findings	Abnormal Findings

Older Adults

Skin Colour and Pigmentation. **Senile lentigines** are commonly called "liver spots," and are small, flat, brown macules that are common variations of hyperpigmentation. They appear after extensive sun exposure on the forearms and dorsa of the hands. They are not malignant and require no treatment.

Moisture. Dry skin (xerosis) is common. Dry skin itches and appears flaky and loose.

Texture. Acrochordons, or "skin tags," are overgrowths of normal skin that form a stalk and are polyplike. They occur frequently on eyelids, cheeks, neck, axillae, and trunk.

Thickness. With aging, the skin looks as thin as parchment, and the subcutaneous fat diminishes. Thinner skin is evident over the dorsa of the hands, forearms, lower legs, dorsa of the feet, and bony prominences.

Aging skin increases risk for pressure ulcers (see Table 5.5).

Hair. Hair growth decreases, and the amount decreases in the axillae and pubic areas. After menopause, women may develop bristly hairs on the chin or upper lip as a result of unopposed androgens.

In men, coarse terminal hairs develop in the ears, nose, and eyebrows, although the beard is unchanged. Male pattern balding, or alopecia, is a genetic trait. It is usually a gradual receding of the anterior hairline in a symmetrical W shape.

In men and women, scalp hair gradually turns grey because of a decrease in melanocyte function.

Nails. Nail growth rate decreases, and local injuries in the nail matrix may produce longitudinal ridges. The surface may be brittle or peeling and sometimes yellowed. Toenails also are thickened and may grow misshapen, almost grotesque. The thickening may be a process of aging, or it may be caused by chronic peripheral vascular disease.

Fungal infections are common in aging, with thickened, crumbling toenails and erythematous scaling on contiguous skin surfaces.

Normal Range of Findings	Abnormal Findings
Mobility and Turgor. Turgor is decreased (less elasticity), and the skin recedes slowly or "tents" and stands by itself.	

For more information on assessment of skin, hair, and nails, see Chapter 13 in *Jarvis: Physical Examination and Health Assessment,* 3rd Canadian edition, page 228.

TEACH SKIN SELF-EXAMINATION

Teach all adults to examine their skin once a month, using the ABCDE rule (see page 39), to detect warning signals of any suspect lesions. They should use a well-lighted room that has a full-length mirror. It helps to have a small handheld mirror. They should ask a relative to search skin areas difficult to see (e.g., behind ears, back of neck, back). They should follow the sequence outlined below and report any suspicious lesions promptly to an appropriate health care provided.

1. Undress completely. Check forearms, palms, space between fingers. Turn over hands and study the backs.
2. Face mirror; bend arms at elbows. Study arms in mirror.
3. Face mirror and study entire front of body. Start at face, neck, torso, working down to lower legs.
4. Pivot to right side facing mirror. Study sides of upper arms, working down to ankles. Repeat with left side.
5. With back to mirror, study buttocks, thighs, lower legs.
6. Use handheld mirror to study upper back.
7. Use handheld mirror to study scalp, lifting the hair. A blow-dryer on a cool setting helps to lift hair.
8. Sit on chair or bed. Study insides of each leg and soles of feet. Use small mirror to help.

Summary Checklist: Skin, Hair, and Nails

1. **Inspect the skin:**
   Colour
   General pigmentation
   Areas of hypopigmentation or hyperpigmentation
   Abnormal colour changes
2. **Palpate the skin:**
   Temperature
   Moisture

   Texture
   Thickness
   Edema
   Mobility and turgor
   Hygiene
   Vascularity or bruising
3. **Note any lesions:**
   Colour
   Shape and configuration

Size
Location and distribution on body
4. **Inspect and palpate the hair:**
Texture
Distribution
Any scalp lesions

5. **Inspect and palpate the nails:**
Shape and contour
Consistency
Colour
6. **Teach skin self-examination and health promotion**

ABNORMAL FINDINGS

TABLE 5.1	Detecting Colour Changes in Light and Dark Skin	
Cause	**Note Appearance**	
	Light Skin	*Dark Skin*
Pallor		
Anemia: decreased hematocrit	Generalized pallor	Brown skin appears yellow-brown, dull; black skin appears ashen grey, dull; skin loses its healthy glow
Shock: decreased perfusion, vasoconstriction		Check areas with least pigmentation, such as conjunctivae and mucous membranes.
Local arterial insufficiency	Marked localized pallor (e.g., lower extremities, especially when elevated)	Ashen grey, dull; cool to palpation
Albinism: total absence of pigment melanin throughout the integument	Whitish pink	Tan, cream, white
Vitiligo: patchy depigmentation from destruction of melanocytes	Patchy milky white spots, often symmetrical bilaterally	Same as for light skin
Cyanosis		
Increased amount of unoxygenated hemoglobin	Dusky blue	Dark but dull, lifeless; only severe cyanosis is apparent in skin. Check conjunctivae, oral mucosa, and nail beds.
Central: chronic heart and lung disease causes arterial desaturation	Grey colouration	Dark but dull, lifeless; only severe cyanosis is apparent in skin
Peripheral: exposure to cold, anxiety	Nail beds dusky	Hard to detect

TABLE 5.1	Detecting Colour Changes in Light and Dark Skin—cont'd	
Cause	**Note Appearance**	
	Light Skin	*Dark Skin*
Erythema		
Hyperemia: increased blood flow through engorged arterioles, such as in inflammation, fever, alcohol intake, blushing	Red, bright pink	Purplish tinge, but difficult to see Palpate for increased warmth with inflammation, for taut skin, and for hardening of deep tissues.
Polycythemia: increased number of red blood cells, capillary stasis	Ruddy blue in face, oral mucosa, conjunctiva, hands, and feet	Well concealed by pigment Check for redness in lips.
Carbon monoxide poisoning	Bright cherry red in face and upper torso	Cherry-red colour in nail beds, lips, and oral mucosa
Venous stasis: decreased blood flow from area, engorged venules	Dusky rubor of dependent extremities; a prelude to necrosis with pressure sore	Easily masked Palpate for warmth or edema.
Jaundice		
Increased serum bilirubin (>2 to 3 mg/100 mL) due to liver inflammation or hemolytic disease, such as postsevere burn state or some infections	Yellow in sclera, hard palate, mucous membranes, then over skin	Check sclera for yellow near limbus; do not mistake normal yellowish fatty deposits in the periphery under the eyelids for jaundice; jaundice is best noted in junction of hard and soft palate and also palms.
Carotenemia: increased serum carotene from ingestion of large amounts of carotene-rich foods	Yellow-orange in forehead, palms and soles, and nasolabial folds, but no yellowing in sclera or mucous membranes	Yellow-orange tinge in palms and soles
Uremia: in renal failure, urochrome pigments are retained in the blood	Orange-green or grey overlying pallor of anemia; ecchymoses and purpura may also be present	Easily masked Rely on laboratory and clinical findings.
Brown-Tan		
Addison's disease: cortisol deficiency stimulates increased melanin production	Bronzed appearance, an "eternal tan," most apparent around nipples, perineum, genitalia, and pressure points (inner thighs, buttocks, elbows, axillae)	Easily masked Rely on laboratory and clinical findings.
Café-au-lait spots: caused by increased melanin pigment in basal cell layer	Tan to light brown, irregularly shaped, oval patches with well-defined borders	

TABLE 5.2   Common Shapes and Configurations of Skin Lesions

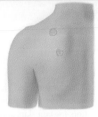

ANNULAR: circular lesions that begin in centre and spread to periphery (e.g., tinea corporis [ringworm], tinea versicolor, pityriasis rosea)

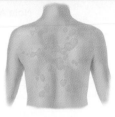

CONFLUENT: lesions that run together (e.g., urticaria [hives])

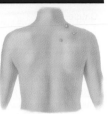

DISCRETE: distinct, individual lesions that remain separate (e.g., molluscum)

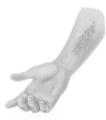

GROUPED: clusters of lesions (e.g., vesicles of contact dermatitis)

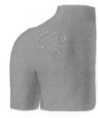

GYRATE: twisted, coiled, spiral, or snakelike lesions

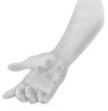

TARGET (IRIS): lesions that resemble iris of eye; concentric rings of colour in the lesions (e.g., erythema multiforme)

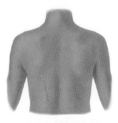

LINEAR: lesions form a scratch, streak, line, or stripe

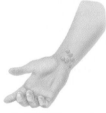

POLYCYCLIC: annular lesions that grow together (e.g., lichen planus, psoriasis)

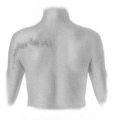

ZOSTERIFORM: lesions form a linear arrangement along a nerve route (e.g., herpes zoster)

TABLE 5.3   Primary Skin Lesions*

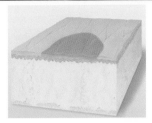

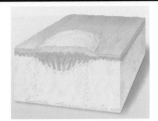

MACULE: Solely a colour change; flat and circumscribed, <1 cm diameter
Examples: freckle, flat nevi, hypopigmentation, petechiae, measles, scarlet fever
PATCH: Macules >1 cm diameter
Examples: Mongolian spot, vitiligo, café au lait spot, chloasma, measles rash

PAPULE: Solid, elevated, and circumscribed, <1 cm diameter; caused by superficial thickening in the epidermis
Examples: elevated nevus (mole), lichen planus, molluscum, wart (verruca)
PLAQUE: Papules that coalesce to form surface elevation wider than 1 cm containing plateaulike, disc-shaped lesions
Examples: psoriasis, lichen planus

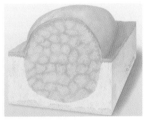

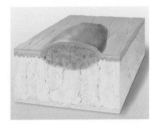

NODULE: Solid, elevated, hard or soft lesion >1 cm diameter; may extend deeper into dermis than papule
Examples: xanthoma, fibroma, intradermal nevi
TUMOUR: Lesion larger than a few centimetres in diameter, firm or soft, deeper into dermis; may be benign or malignant, although "tumour" implies "cancer" to most people
Examples: lipoma, hemangioma

WHEAL: Superficial, raised, transient, and erythematous lesion; slightly irregular shape because of edema (fluid held diffusely in the tissues)
Examples: mosquito bite, allergic reaction, dermographism
URTICARIA (HIVES): Wheals that coalesce to form extensive reaction; intensely pruritic

Continued

TABLE 5.3 Primary Skin Lesions—cont'd

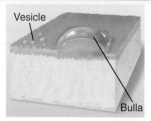

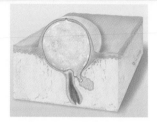

VESICLE (BLISTER): Elevated cavity containing free clear fluid, up to 1 cm; clear serum flows if wall is ruptured

Examples: herpes simplex, early varicella (chicken pox), herpes zoster (shingles), contact dermatitis

BULLA: Usually single-chambered (unilocular); superficial in epidermis; >1 cm diameter thin-walled, so it ruptures easily

Examples: friction blister, pemphigus, burns, contact dermatitis

PUSTULE: Cavity filled with turbid fluid (pus); circumscribed and elevated

Examples: impetigo, acne

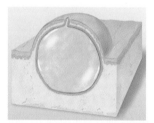

CYST: Encapsulated fluid-filled cavity in dermis or subcutaneous layer, tensely elevating skin

Examples: sebaceous cyst, trichilemmal cyst (wen)

*The immediate result of a specific causative factor; primary lesions develop on previously unaltered skin.
Line drawings © Pat Thomas, 2010.

TABLE 5.4   Secondary Skin Lesions*

Debris on Skin Surface

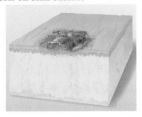

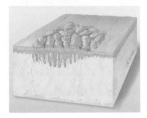

CRUST: Thickened, dried-out exudate left when vesicles or pustules burst or dry up. Colour can be red-brown, honeylike, or yellow, depending on the fluid's ingredients (blood, serum, pus).
Examples: impetigo (dry, honey-coloured), weeping eczematous dermatitis, scab following abrasion

SCALE: Compact, desiccated flakes of skin, dry or greasy, silvery or white, from shedding of dead excess keratin cells
Examples: lesions after scarlet fever or drug reaction (laminated sheets), psoriasis (silver, mica-like), seborrheic dermatitis (yellow, greasy), eczema, ichthyosis (large, adherent, laminated), dry skin

Break in Continuity of Surface

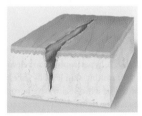

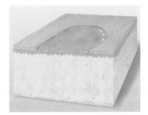

FISSURE: Linear crack with abrupt edges, extending into dermis, dry or moist
Examples: cheilosis (at corners of mouth as a result of excess moisture); athlete's foot

EROSION: Scooped-out but shallow depression; superficial; epidermis lost; moist but no bleeding; healing without scar because erosion does not extend into dermis

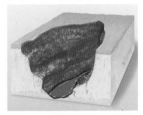

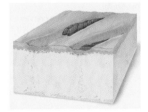

ULCER: Deeper depression extending into dermis, irregular shaped; may bleed; leaves scar when heals
Examples: stasis ulcer, pressure sore, chancre

EXCORIATION: Self-inflicted abrasion; superficial; sometimes crusted; scratches from intense itching
Examples: lesions caused by scratching of insect bites, scabies, dermatitis, varicella

Continued

TABLE 5.4	Secondary Skin Lesions—cont'd

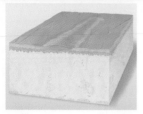

SCAR: Connective tissue (collagen) that replaces normal tissue after a skin lesion is repaired; a permanent fibrotic change
Examples: healed area of surgery or injury, acne

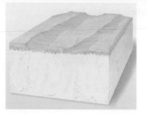

ATROPHIC SCAR: Depression of skin level as a result of loss of tissue; a thinning of the epidermis
Example: striae

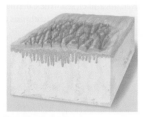

LICHENIFICATION: Thickening of skin with production of tightly packed sets of papules, caused by prolonged intense scratching; looks like surface of moss (or lichen)

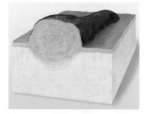

KELOID: A hypertrophic scar; elevation of the resulting skin level by excess scar tissue, which is invasive beyond the site of original injury; may increase long after healing occurs; looks smooth, rubbery, "clawlike"; has a higher incidence among individuals of African descent

Note: Combinations of primary and secondary lesions may co-exist in the same person. Such combined designations may be termed *papulosquamous, maculopapular, vesiculopustular,* or *papulovesicular.*
*Resulting from a change in a primary lesion due to the passage of time; an evolutionary change.
© Pat Thomas, 2010.

TABLE 5.5	Pressure Ulcer (Decubitus Ulcer)

In Canada, the prevalence of pressure ulcers is estimated to be about 4% in an acute care setting compared to 30% in hospital-based complex care environments. These estimates are higher than those in most other countries worldwide, perhaps because of issues regarding length of stay in hospital settings and increasing numbers of people with overall level of illness who present in acute and long-term care environments (Denny, Lawand, & Perry, 2013).

Pressure ulcers appear on the skin over a bony prominence when circulation is impaired. This occurs when a person is confined to bed or is immobilized. Immobilization impedes delivery of blood, which carries oxygen and nutrients to the skin, and it impedes venous drainage, which carries metabolic wastes away from the skin. These impediments result in ischemia and cell death. Common sites for pressure ulcers are on the back (heel, ischium, sacrum, elbow, scapula, and vertebra) and the side (ankle, knee, hip, rib, and shoulder).

Risk factors for pressure ulcers include impaired mobility, thin fragile skin of aging, decreased sensory perception (which causes inability to perceive pain accompanying prolonged pressure), impaired level of consciousness (which causes inability to respond to pain), moisture from urine or stool incontinence, excessive perspiration or wound drainage, shearing injury (being pulled down or across in bed), poor nutrition, and infection. Learning about risk factors and prevention of pressure ulcers are far more easily accomplished than is treatment of existing ulcers. However, once pressure ulcers occur, they are assessed by stage depending on the pressure ulcer depth (National Pressure Ulcer Advisory Panel [NPUAP], 2007):

Stage I
Intact skin appears red but unbroken. Localized redness in lightly pigmented skin will blanch (turns light with pressure). Affected dark skin appears darker but does not blanch.

Stage II
Partial-thickness skin erosion causes loss of epidermis or also the dermis. Superficial ulcer looks shallow, like an abrasion or open blister with a red-pink wound bed.

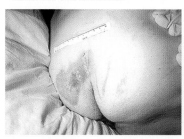

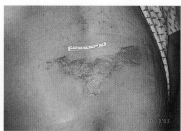

Continued

TABLE 5.5	Pressure Ulcer (Decubitus Ulcer)—cont'd

Stage III

Full-thickness pressure ulcer extends into the subcutaneous tissue and resembles a crater. Subcutaneous fat may be visible, but not muscle, bone, or tendon.

Stage IV

Full-thickness pressure ulcer involves all skin layers and extends into supporting tissue. Exposes muscle, tendon, or bone, and may show slough (stringy matter attached to wound bed) or eschar (black or brown necrotic tissue).

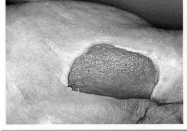
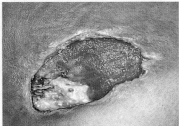

See Illustration Credits for source information.

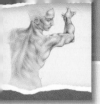

CHAPTER 6

Head, Face, and Neck, Including Regional Lymphatic System

STRUCTURE AND FUNCTION

Facial structures are, in general, symmetrical; the eyebrows, eyes, ears, nose, and mouth appear about the same on both sides. The palpebral fissures—the openings between the eyelids—are equal bilaterally. Also, the nasolabial folds—the creases extending from the nose to each corner of the mouth—should be symmetrical. Facial sensations of pain or touch are mediated by the three sensory branches of cranial nerve V (the trigeminal nerve). The facial expressions are formed by the muscles mediated by cranial nerve VII (the facial nerve).

Two pairs of **salivary glands** are accessible to examination on the face

(Fig. 6.1). The **parotid glands** are in the cheeks over the mandible, anterior to and below the ear. They are the largest of the salivary glands but are not normally palpable. The **submandibular glands** are beneath the mandible at the angle of the jaw. A third pair, the **sublingual glands**, lie in the floor of the mouth. (Salivary gland function is described in Chapter 9.) The **temporal artery** lies superior to the temporalis muscle, and its pulsation is palpable anterior to the ear.

The head and neck have a rich supply of **lymph nodes** (Fig. 6.2). The nodes are small, oval clusters of lymphatic tissue. The nodes filter

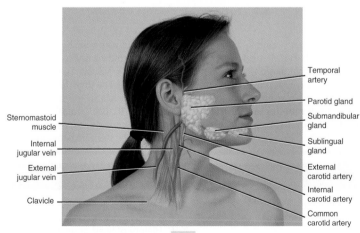

Temporal artery

Parotid gland

Submandibular gland

Sublingual gland

External carotid artery

Internal carotid artery

Common carotid artery

Sternomastoid muscle

Internal jugular vein

External jugular vein

Clavicle

6.1

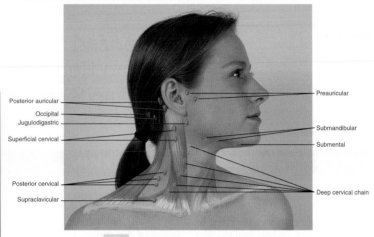

Posterior auricular
Occipital
Jugulodigastric
Superficial cervical
Posterior cervical
Supraclavicular
Preauricular
Submandibular
Submental
Deep cervical chain

6.2 Lymph nodes of the head and neck.

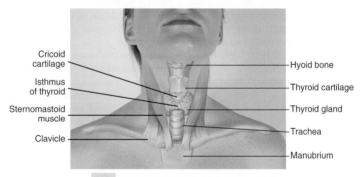

Cricoid cartilage
Isthmus of thyroid
Sternomastoid muscle
Clavicle
Hyoid bone
Thyroid cartilage
Thyroid gland
Trachea
Manubrium

6.3 Landmarks and structures in the neck.

the lymph and engulf pathogens, preventing harmful substances from entering the circulation.

The neck contains many structures lying in close proximity (Fig. 6.3). The major **neck muscles** are the **sternomastoid** and the **trapezius** on the upper back. The carotid artery and internal jugular vein lie beneath the sternomastoid muscle. (Assessment of the neck vessels is discussed in Chapter 12.) The **thyroid gland** straddles the trachea in the middle of the neck, and its two conical lobes each curve posteriorly between the trachea and the sternomastoid muscle.

SUBJECTIVE DATA

1. Headache
2. Head injury
3. Dizziness
4. Neck pain, limitation of motion
5. Lumps or swelling
6. History of head or neck surgery

OBJECTIVE DATA

Normal Range of Findings	Abnormal Findings

The Head

Inspect and Palpate the Skull

Size and Shape. Normocephalic describes a round, symmetrical skull appropriately related to body size.

The skull normally feels symmetrical and smooth. The cranial bones with normal protrusions are the forehead, the lateral edge of each parietal bone, the occipital bone, and the mastoid process behind each ear. There is no tenderness on palpation.

Temporal Area. Palpate the temporal artery above the zygomatic (cheek) bone between the eye and top of the ear.

Palpate the temporomandibular joint (located just below the temporal artery and anterior to the tragus) as the patient opens the mouth; normal movement is smooth, with no limitation or tenderness.

Inspect the Face

Facial Structures. Note the facial expression and its appropriateness for behaviour or reported mood. Anxiety is common in hospitalized or ill patients. Note symmetry of eyebrows, palpebral fissures, nasolabial folds, and sides of the mouth. Note any abnormal facial structures (coarse facial features, exophthalmos, changes in skin colour or pigmentation), and any abnormal swelling. Also note any involuntary movements (tics) in the facial muscles. Normally, there are none.

Abnormal Findings column:

Deformities: microcephaly (abnormally small head); macrocephaly (abnormally large head), caused by hydrocephaly, or acromegaly.

Lumps, depressions, or abnormal protrusions.

With **temporal arteritis**, the artery looks more tortuous and feels hardened and tender.

Crepitation, limited range of motion (ROM), or tenderness.

Hostility or aggression. Tense, rigid muscles may indicate anxiety or pain; a flat affect may indicate depression.

Marked asymmetry may be seen with central brain lesion (e.g., brain attack) or with peripheral damage to cranial nerve VII (Bell's palsy). (See Table 14.4, p. 297, in Jarvis: *Physical Examination and Health Assessment,* 3rd Canadian edition.) Edema in the face occurs first around the eyes (periorbital) and the cheeks, where the subcutaneous tissue is relatively loose.

Note grinding of jaws, tics or fasciculations, and excessive blinking.

Continued

Normal Range of Findings	Abnormal Findings

The Neck

Inspect and Palpate the Neck

Symmetry. Head position is centred in the midline, and the accessory neck muscles should be symmetrical.

Head tilt occurs with muscle spasm. Head and neck rigidity occurs with arthritis.

Note pain at any particular movement.

Range of Motion. Ask the patient to touch the chin to the chest, turn the head to the right and left, try to touch each ear to the shoulder (without elevating shoulders), and to extend the head backward. When the neck is supple, motion is smooth and controlled.

Note ratchety movement or limited movement, which may be due to cervical arthritis or inflammation of neck muscles. With arthritis, the neck is rigid and the patient turns at the shoulders rather than at the neck.

Lymph Nodes. Using a gentle circular motion of your fingertips and beginning with the preauricular lymph nodes in front of the ear, palpate the 10 groups of lymph nodes in a routine order. Be systematic and thorough. Use gentle pressure because strong pressure could push the nodes into the neck muscles. It is usually most efficient to palpate with both hands, comparing the two sides for symmetry.

If any nodes are palpable, note their location, size, shape, delimitation (discrete or clumped together), mobility, consistency, and tenderness. Cervical nodes often are palpable in healthy persons, although this palpability decreases with age. Normal nodes feel movable, discrete, soft, and nontender. If nodes are enlarged or tender, check the area they drain for the source of the problem. For example, enlargement or tenderness of those in the upper cervical or submandibular area is often related to inflammation or a neoplasm in the head and neck. Follow up on your findings, or refer your patient to a specialist. An enlarged lymph node necessitates prompt attention, particularly when you cannot find the source of the problem.

Lymphadenopathy is disease of the lymph nodes with enlargement to >1 cm from infection, allergy, or neoplasm.

The following are commonly associated with **lymphadenopathy** (enlargement of the lymph nodes >1 cm) but are not definitive in all circumstances:

- Acute infection: Nodes are bilateral, enlarged, warm, tender, and firm but freely movable.
- Chronic inflammation Nodes are clumped (e.g., in tuberculosis).
- Cancerous nodes: Nodes are hard, unilateral, nontender, and fixed.
- Human immunodeficiency virus (HIV) infection: Nodes are enlarged, firm, nontender, and mobile. Occipital node lymphadenopathy is common.
- Neoplasm in the thorax or abdomen: A single left node (Virchow's node) may be enlarged, nontender, and hard.
- Hodgkin's lymphoma: Discrete nodes that are painless and rubbery gradually appear.

Normal Range of Findings	Abnormal Findings

Thyroid Gland. Position a standing lamp to shine tangentially across the neck to highlight any possible swelling. Supply the patient with a glass of water, and first inspect the neck as the patient takes a sip and swallows. Thyroid tissue normally moves up with a swallow.

To palpate the thyroid using a posterior approach, move behind the person (Fig. 6.4). Ask him or her to sit up very straight and then to bend the head slightly forward and to the right. This will relax the neck muscles. Use the fingers of your left hand to push the trachea slightly to the right.

Curve your right fingers between the trachea and the sternomastoid muscle, retracting it slightly, and ask the patient to take a sip of water. The thyroid moves up under your fingers with the trachea and larynx as the patient swallows. Reverse the procedure for the left side.

Usually, you cannot palpate a normal adult thyroid. In some patients who have a long, thin neck, you can feel the isthmus over the tracheal rings. The lateral lobes usually are not palpable; check them for enlargement, consistency, symmetry, and the presence of nodules.

Abnormalities include enlarged lobes that are easily palpated before swallowing or that are tender on palpation and the presence of nodules or lumps. (See Table 14.3, p. 296, in Jarvis: *Physical Examination and Health Assessment,* 3rd Canadian edition.)

Continued

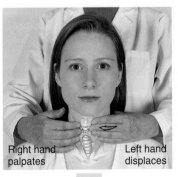

Right hand palpates   Left hand displaces

6.4

Normal Range of Findings	Abnormal Findings

DEVELOPMENTAL CONSIDERATIONS

Infants and Children. An infant's **head size** is measured with measuring tape at each visit up to age 2 years, then yearly up to age 6 years. (Measurement of head circumference is described in detail in Chapter 4.)

Gently palpate the skull and **fontanelles** while the infant is calm and somewhat in a sitting position (crying, lying down, or vomiting may cause the anterior fontanelle to look full and bulging). The skull should feel smooth and fused except at the fontanelles. The fontanelles feel firm, slightly concave, and well defined against the edges of the cranial bones. You may see slight arterial pulsations in the anterior fontanelle.

The posterior fontanelle may not be palpable at birth. If it is, it measures 1 cm and closes by 1 to 2 months. The anterior fontanelle may be small at birth and enlarges to 2.5 cm × 2.5 cm. A large diameter of 4 to 5 cm occasionally may be normal in infants younger than 6 months. A small fontanelle usually is normal.

The anterior fontanelle closes between 9 months and 2 years. Early closure may be insignificant if head growth proceeds normally.

During infancy, cervical lymph nodes are not normally palpable, but a child's lymph nodes are; they feel more prominent than an adult's until after puberty, when lymphoid tissue begins to atrophy. Palpable nodes <3 mm are normal. They may be up to 1 cm in size in the cervical and inguinal areas but are discrete, move easily, and are nontender. Children have a higher incidence of infection, and so you will expect a greater incidence of inflammatory adenopathy among children. No other mass should occur in the neck.

Microcephalic: Head size is below norms for age.

Macrocephalic: Head is large for age or rapidly increasing in size (e.g., as in hydrocephalus [increased cerebrospinal fluid]).

A true tense or bulging fontanelle occurs with acute increased intracranial pressure.

Depressed and sunken fontanelles occur with dehydration or malnutrition.

Pulsations may be markedly noticeable with increased intracranial pressure.

Delayed closure or larger than normal fontanelles occur with hydrocephalus, Down syndrome, hypothyroidism, or rickets.

A small fontanelle may be a sign of microcephaly, as is early closure.

Cervical nodes >1 cm are considered enlarged.

Thyroglossal duct cyst is a cystic lump high up in the midline that is freely movable and that rises up during swallowing.

Supraclavicular nodes enlarge with Hodgkin's disease.

Normal Range of Findings	Abnormal Findings
Pregnant Women. The thyroid gland may be normally palpable during the second trimester; chloasma may show on the face. This is a blotchy, hyperpigmented area over the cheeks and forehead that fades after delivery.	
Older Adults. In some older adults, a mild rhythmic tremor of the head is normal. **Senile tremors** are benign and include head nodding (as if saying yes or no) and tongue protrusion.	
If some teeth have been lost, the lower face looks unusually small, with the mouth sunken in.	
The neck may show an increased cervical concave (or inward) curve when the head and jaw are extended forward to compensate for kyphosis of the spine. During the examination, direct the older adult to perform ROM slowly; he or she may experience dizziness with side movements.	

For more information on assessment of the head and neck, see Chapter 14 in Jarvis: *Physical Examination and Health Assessment,* 3rd Canadian edition, pages 279.

Summary Checklist: Head, Face, and Neck, Including Examination of Regional Lymphatic System

1. **Inspect and palpate the skull:**
   General size and contour
   Any deformities, lumps, tenderness
   Palpation of temporal artery, temporomandibular joint
2. **Inspect the face:**
   Facial expression
   Symmetry of movement (cranial nerve VII)
   Any involuntary movements, edema, lesions
3. **Inspect and palpate the neck:**
   Active ROM
   Enlargement of salivary glands, lymph nodes, thyroid gland
4. **Auscultate the thyroid (if enlarged) for bruit**
5. **Engage in teaching and health promotion**

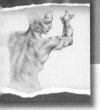

CHAPTER 7

Eyes

STRUCTURE AND FUNCTION

The eye is the sensory organ of vision. The **eyelids** protect the eye from injury, strong light, and dust (Fig. 7.1). The **palpebral fissure** is the elliptical open space between the eyelids.

The exposed part of the eye has a transparent protective covering, the **conjunctiva.** The *palpebral* conjunctiva lines the eyelids and is clear, with many small blood vessels. It forms a deep recess and then folds back over the eye. The *bulbar* conjunctiva overlays the eyeball, with the white sclera showing through. At the limbus, the conjunctiva merges with the cornea. The **cornea** covers and protects the iris and pupil.

The eye is a sphere composed of three concentric coats: (a) the outer fibrous **sclera,** (b) the middle vascular **choroid,** and (c) the inner nervous **retina** (Fig. 7.2). Inside the retina is the transparent vitreous body.

The retina is the visual receptive layer of the eye in which light waves are changed into nerve impulses. The **ocular fundus** is the area of the retina visible through the ophthalmoscope (Fig. 7.3).

The **optic disc** (or *optic papilla*) is the area in which fibres from the retina converge to form the optic nerve. The **macula** is the area of sharpest vision.

SOCIAL DETERMINANTS OF HEALTH CONSIDERATIONS

Many people in Canada cannot afford vision care costs, including vision

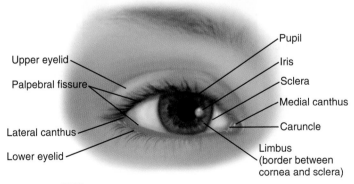

7.1 External eye structures. *(© Pat Thomas, 2006.)*

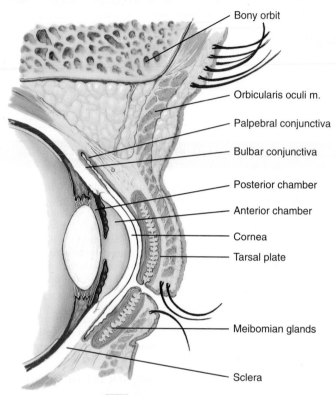

Bony orbit

Orbicularis oculi m.

Palpebral conjunctiva

Bulbar conjunctiva

Posterior chamber

Anterior chamber

Cornea

Tarsal plate

Meibomian glands

Sclera

7.2 Internal eye structures.

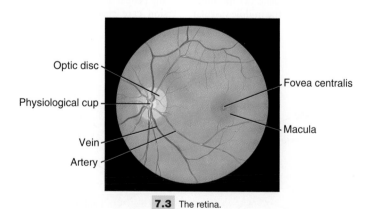

Optic disc

Physiological cup

Vein

Artery

Fovea centralis

Macula

7.3 The retina.

testing, eye exams, glasses, or contact lenses (Jin & Trope, 2011). Provincial health care plans typically only provide coverage for eye examinations for children up to age 18 years and adults over age 65 (Canadian Ophthalmological Society Clinical Practice Guideline Expert Committee [COSCPGEC], 2007, page 41). Eye glasses are not covered in any of the provinces for any age. Nurses working in community and acute care need to consider the effect of low income on access to routine eye care and the ability to pay for corrective lenses. People who cannot afford vision testing or corrective lenses must be referred to agencies that can provide those services free of charge or at a reduced cost.

SUBJECTIVE DATA

1. Vision difficulty (decreased acuity, blurring, blind spots)
2. Pain
3. Strabismus, diplopia
4. Redness, swelling
5. Watering, discharge
6. History of ocular problems
7. Glaucoma
8. Use of glasses or contact lenses
9. Self-care behaviours (vision last tested, method of care for contacts or glasses, efforts to protect eyes)

OBJECTIVE DATA

EQUIPMENT NEEDED

Snellen eye chart
Handheld visual screener
Opaque card or occluder

Penlight
Applicator stick
Ophthalmoscope

Normal Range of Findings	Abnormal Findings
Test Central Visual Acuity	
Snellen Eye Chart	
Position the patient on a mark exactly 20 feet (6.1 m) from the chart. If the patient wears glasses or contact lenses, leave them on. Shield one eye at a time with an opaque card during the test. Ask the patient to read through the chart to the smallest line of letters possible.	Note hesitancy, squinting, leaning forward, and misreading letters.

Continued

Normal Range of Findings	Abnormal Findings

Record the result using the numerical fraction at the end of the last successful line read. Indicate whether the patient missed any letters or whether corrective lenses were worn: for example, "O.D.* 20/30-1, with glasses."

Normal visual acuity is 20/20. The top number (numerator) indicates the distance the patient is standing from the chart; the bottom number (denominator) is the distance at which a normal eye could have read that particular line.

The larger the denominator, the poorer the vision. If vision is poorer than 20/30, refer to an ophthalmologist or optometrist. Vision may be impaired as a result of refractive error, opacity in the media (cornea, lens, vitreous), or disorder in the retina or optic pathway.

Near Vision

For patients older than 40 years or for those who report increasing difficulty reading, test near vision with a hand-held vision screener with various sizes of print (e.g., a Jaeger card). Instruct the patient to hold the card in good light about 14 inches (35 cm) from the eye. Test each eye separately, with glasses on. A normal result is "14/14" in each eye, reading without hesitancy and without moving the card closer or farther away.

If the patient moves the card farther away, this is a possible sign of **presbyopia,** the decrease in power of accommodation with aging.

Test Visual Fields

Confrontation Test

Position yourself at eye level with the patient, about 60 cm away. Direct the patient to cover one eye with an opaque card and to look straight at you with the other eye. Cover your own eye opposite to the patient's covered one. Hold a pencil or your flicking finger as a target midline between you and the patient, at the periphery of vision, and slowly advance it inward from the periphery in several directions (upward, downward, temporally, nasally).

*O.D., *oculus dexter,* or right eye.

Normal Range of Findings	Abnormal Findings

Ask the patient to say, "Now" when he or she first sees the target; this location should be the same as when you also see the object.

If the patient is unable to see the object as you do, the test result suggests peripheral field loss. Refer the patient to an optometrist or ophthalmologist for more precise testing with a tangent screen.

Inspect Extraocular Muscle Function

Diagnostic Positions Test

Leading the eyes through the six cardinal positions of gaze reveals any muscle weakness during movement. Ask the patient to hold the head steady and follow the movement of your finger, pen, or penlight only with the eyes. Hold the target object back about 30 cm so the patient can focus on it comfortably, and move it to each of the six positions, hold it momentarily, then move it back to centre. Progress clockwise (Fig. 7.4). A normal response is parallel tracking of the object with both eyes.

Eye movement that is not parallel is abnormal. Failure to follow in a certain direction indicates weakness of an extraocular muscle (EOM) or dysfunction of the cranial nerve that innervates it.

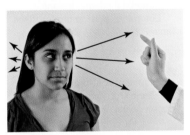

7.4 Diagnostics positions test.

In addition to parallel movement, note any **nystagmus,** a fine oscillating movement best seen around the iris. Mild nystagmus at extreme lateral gaze is normal; nystagmus at any other position is not.

Finally, note that the upper eyelid continues to overlap the superior part of the iris, even during downward movement.

Nystagmus occurs with disease of the semicircular canals in the ears, a paretic eye muscle, multiple sclerosis, or brain lesions.

A white rim of sclera between the eyelid and the iris, referred to as "lid lag," occurs with hyperthyroidism.

Continued

Normal Range of Findings	Abnormal Findings

Inspect External Ocular Structures

General

Note the patient's ability to move around the room with vision functioning well enough to avoid obstacles and respond to your directions. The facial expression is relaxed with adequate vision.

Groping with hands.
Squinting or craning forward.

Eyebrows

Normally, the eyebrows are present bilaterally, move symmetrically as the facial expression changes, and have no scaling or lesions.

Absence of lateral third of brow occurs with hypothyroidism.
Unequal or absent movement with nerve damage.
Scaling with seborrhea.

Eyelids and Lashes

The upper eyelids normally overlap the superior part of the iris and approximate completely when closed. The skin is intact, without redness, swelling, discharge, or lesions.
The palpebral fissures are horizontal or slightly upward in some people of East Asian descent.
The eyelashes are evenly distributed along the eyelid margins and curve outward.

Lid lag occurs with hyperthyroidism. Incomplete closure creates risk for corneal damage.

Ptosis: drooping of upper lid, as with myasthenia gravis.
Periorbital edema, lesions.
Ectropion and entropion (see Table 7.2).

Eyeballs

The eyeballs are aligned normally in their sockets with no protrusion or sunken appearance. Some people of African descent may have a slight protrusion of the eyeball beyond the supraorbital ridge.

Exophthalmos (protruding eyes; see Table 7.2) and enophthalmos (sunken eyes).

Normal Range of Findings	Abnormal Findings

Conjunctiva and Sclera

Ask the patient to look up. Using your thumbs, slide the patient's lower eyelids down along the bony orbital rim. Take care not to push against the eyeball. Inspect the exposed area. The eyeball looks moist and glossy. Numerous small blood vessels normally show through the transparent conjunctiva. Otherwise, the conjunctivae are clear and show the normal colour of the structure below: pink over the lower lids and white over the sclera. Note any colour change, swelling, or lesions.

General reddening.
Cyanosis of the lower lids.
Pallor near the outer canthus of the lower eyelid (may indicate anemia; the inner canthus normally contains less pigmentation).

The sclera is china white, although in people with dark skin, it is occasionally grey-blue or "muddy." Dark-skinned people may have small brown macules (like freckles) on the sclera; do not confuse these with foreign bodies or petechiae. Some people with dark skin may have yellowish fatty deposits beneath the lids away from the cornea. Do not confuse these yellow spots with the overall scleral yellowing that accompanies jaundice.

Scleral icterus (an even yellowing of the sclera extending up to the cornea), indicative of jaundice.
Tenderness, foreign body, discharge, or lesions.

Inspect Anterior Eyeball Structures

Cornea and Lens

Shine a light from the side across the patient's cornea, and check for smoothness and clarity. There should be no opacities (cloudiness) in the cornea, in the anterior chamber, or in the lens behind the pupil. Do not confuse an *arcus senilis* with an opacity. This is a normal finding in older adults and is described on p. 76.

A corneal abrasion causes irregular ridges in reflected light, producing a shattered appearance with light rays.

Continued

Normal Range of Findings	Abnormal Findings

Iris and Pupils

The iris normally appears flat, with a round regular shape and even colouration. Normally, the pupils appear round, regular, and of equal size in both eyes. In adults, resting size is from 3 to 5 mm. A small number of people (5%) normally have pupils of two different sizes, which is termed **anisocoria.**

Irregular shape.
Although they may be normal, unequal-sized pupils necessitate investigation for central nervous system injury.

To test the **pupillary light reflex,** darken the room and ask the patient to gaze into the distance. (This dilates the pupils.) Advance a light in from the side,* and note the response. Normally you will see (a) constriction of the same-sided pupil (a *direct light reflex*), and (b) simultaneous constriction of the other pupil (a *consensual light reflex*).

Dilated pupils.
Dilated and fixed pupils.
Constricted pupils.
Unequal or no response to light (see Table 7.3).

Test for **accommodation** by asking the patient to focus on a distant object. This process dilates the pupils. Then have the patient shift the gaze to a near object, such as your finger held about 7 to 8 cm from the nose. A normal response includes: (a) pupillary constriction, and (b) convergence of the axes of the eyes.

Absence of constriction or convergence.
Asymmetrical response.

Record the normal response to all these manoeuvres as PERRLA (**p**upils **e**qual, **r**ound, **r**eact to **l**ight, and **a**ccommodation).

Inspect the Ocular Fundus

Darken the room to help dilate the pupils. Remove your own eyeglasses and the patient's because they obstruct close movement; you can compensate for their correction by using the dioptre setting. Contact lenses can be left in.

---

*Always advance the light in from the *side* to test the light reflex. If you advance from the front, the pupils will constrict to accommodate for near vision. Thus, you do not know what the pure response to the light would have been.

Normal Range of Findings	Abnormal Findings

Select the large round aperture with the white light of the ophthalmoscope for routine examination. If the pupils are small, use the smaller white light.

Instruct the patient to keep looking at a light switch (or mark) on the wall across the room, even though your head will get in the way. Staring at a distant, fixed object helps dilate the pupils and hold the retinal structures still.

Match sides with the patient; that is, hold the ophthalmoscope in your *right* hand up to your *right* eye to view the patient's *right* eye (Fig. 7.5, *A* and *B*). You must do this to avoid bumping noses during the procedure. Place your free hand on the patient's shoulder or forehead.

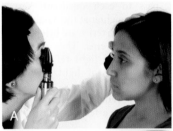
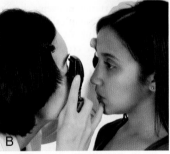

7.5

Systematically inspect the structures in the ocular fundus: (a) optic disc, (b) retinal vessels, (c) general background, and (d) macula (see Fig. 7.3). (Note that the illustration shows a large area of the fundus. Your actual view through the ophthalmoscope is much smaller: slightly larger than 1 disc diameter [DD].)

Optic Disc

The most prominent landmark is the optic disc, located on the nasal side of the retina. Explore these characteristics:

1. **Colour:** Creamy yellow-orange to pink
2. **Shape:** Round or oval
3. **Margins:** Distinct and sharply demarcated, although the nasal edge may be slightly fuzzy.
4. **Cup-disc ratio:** Distinctness varies. When visible, the physiological cup is a brighter yellow-white than rest of the disc. Its width is not more than one-half of the DD.

Pallor.
Hyperemia.
Irregular.
Blurred margins.

Cup extending to the disc border. (See Table 15.9, p. 346, in Jarvis: *Physical Examination and Health Assessment,* 3rd Canadian edition.)

Continued

Normal Range of Findings	Abnormal Findings

Retinal Vessels

Follow a paired artery and vein out to the periphery in the four quadrants (see Fig. 7.3), noting these points:

1. **Number:** A paired artery and vein pass to each quadrant. Vessels look straighter at the nasal side.

   Absence of major vessels.

2. **Colour:** Arteries are brighter red than are veins. They also have the arterial light reflex, with a thin stripe of light down the middle.

3. **Artery–vein ratio:** The ratio comparing the artery-to-vein width is 2:3 or 4:5.

   Arteries too constricted.
   Veins dilated.

4. **Calibre:** Arteries and veins show a regular decrease in calibre as they extend to periphery.

   Focal constriction.
   Neovascularization.

5. **Arteriovenous crossing:** An artery and vein may cross paths. This is not significant if within 2 DD of disc and if no sign of interruption in blood flow is seen. There should be no indenting or displacing of vessel.

   Crossings more than 2 DD away from disc.
   Nicking or pinching of underlying vessel.
   Vessel engorged peripheral to crossing.

6. **Tortuosity:** Mild vessel twisting when present in both eyes is usually congenital and not significant.

   Extreme tortuosity or marked asymmetry in two eyes.

7. **Pulsations:** Visible in veins near the disc as their drainage meets the intermittent pressure of arterial systole (often hard to see).

   Absence of pulsations. (See Table 15.9, p. 346, in Jarvis: *Physical Examination and Health Assessment,* 2nd Canadian edition.)

General Background of the Fundus

The colour normally varies from light red to dark brown-red, generally corresponding to the patient's skin colour. There should be no lesions obstructing the retinal structures.

   Abnormal lesions: hemorrhages, exudates, microaneurysms.

Normal Range of Findings	Abnormal Findings

Macula

The macula is 1 DD in size and is located 2 DD temporal to the disc. Inspect this area last in the funduscopic examination. A bright light on this area of central vision causes some watering, discomfort, and pupillary constriction. Note that the normal colour of the area is somewhat darker than the rest of the fundus, but even and homogeneous. Clumped pigment may occur with aging.

Clumped pigment occurs with trauma or retinal detachment.

Hemorrhage or exudate in the macula occurs with age-related macular degeneration (AMD).

❖ DEVELOPMENTAL CONSIDERATIONS

Infants and Children

With a newborn, test **light perception** using the blink reflex; neonates blink in response to bright light. The pupillary light reflex also shows that the pupils constrict in response to light.

Testing for **strabismus** (squint, crossed eye) is an important screening measure during early childhood. Early recognition and treatment are essential. Diagnosis after age 6 years has a poor prognosis.

Check the **corneal light reflex** by shining a light toward the child's eyes. The light should be reflected at exactly the same spot in the two corneas. Some asymmetry (where one light falls off centre) under age 6 months is normal. Many infants have an *epicanthal fold,* an excess skinfold extending over the inner corner of the eye, partly or totally overlapping the inner canthus. It is present in many children of Eastern Asian descent and in some people of European descent. In some children, the epicanthal folds disappear as they grow, usually by 10 years of age. While they are present, epicanthal folds give a false appearance of malalignment, termed **pseudostrabismus,** but the corneal light reflex is symmetrical.

Absence of blinking.
Absence of pupillary light reflex, especially after 3 weeks, indicates blindness.

Untreated strabismus can lead to permanent visual damage. The resulting loss of vision from disuse is amblyopia ex anopsia.

Asymmetry in the corneal light reflex after 6 months is abnormal and must be investigated.

Continued

Normal Range of Findings	Abnormal Findings
Infants of Eastern Asian descent normally have an upward slant of the palpebral fissures. *Entropion,* a turning inward of the eyelid, is normally found in some children of Eastern Asian descent. If the lashes do not abrade the corneas, it is not significant.	An upward lateral slope together with epicanthal folds and hypertelorism (abnormally wide spacing between the eyes) occurs with Down syndrome.

Older Adults

The eyebrows may show a loss of the outer one-third to one-half of hair because of a decrease in hair follicles. The remaining brow hair is coarse. Because of atrophy of elastic tissues, the skin around the eyes may show wrinkles or crow's feet. The upper lid may be so elongated as to rest on the lashes, a condition called *pseudoptosis* (see Table 7.1).

The eyes may appear sunken from atrophy of the orbital fat. The orbital fat may also herniate, causing bulging at the lower lids and inner third of the upper lids.

Ectropion (lower eyelid dropping away) and entropion (lower eyelid turning in) (see Table 7.2).

The lacrimal apparatus may decrease tear production, causing the eyes to look dry and lustreless, and the patient to feel a burning sensation. **Pingueculae** commonly show on the sclera (see Table 7.1).

Distinguish pinguecula from the abnormal **pterygium,** which is also an opacity on the bulbar conjunctiva, but grows over the cornea and may block vision.

These yellowish elevated nodules are caused by a thickening of the bulbar conjunctiva as a result of prolonged exposure to sun, wind, and dust. Pingueculae appear at the 3:00 and 9:00 positions, first on the nasal side, then on the temporal side.

The cornea may look cloudy with age. **Arcus senilis** is commonly seen around the cornea (see Table 7.1). This is a grey-white arc or circle around the limbus caused by deposition of lipid material. As more lipid accumulates, the cornea may look thickened and raised, but the arcus has no effect on vision.

Xanthelasma are soft, raised, yellow plaques occurring on the eyelids at the inner canthus (see Table 7.1). These commonly occur around the fifth decade of life and are more frequent in women. Xanthelasma occur with both high and normal blood levels of cholesterol and have no pathological significance.

Normal Range of Findings	Abnormal Findings
Pupils are small, and the pupillary light reflex may be slowed. The lens loses transparency and looks opaque. In the ocular fundus, the blood vessels look pale, narrow, and attenuated. Arterioles appear pale and straight with a narrow light reflex. More arteriovenous crossing defects occur.	
A normal development on the retinal surface is **drusen,** or benign degenerative hyaline deposits. They are small, round, yellow dots that are scattered haphazardly on the retina. Although they do not occur in a pattern, drusen are usually symmetrically placed in the two eyes. They have no effect on vision.	Drusen are easily confused with *hard exudates,* an abnormal finding that occurs with a more circular or linear pattern. (See Table 15.10, p. 348, in Jarvis: *Physical Examination and Health Assessment,* 3rd Canadian edition.) Also, drusen in the macular area occur with AMD.

Summary Checklist: Eye Examination

1. **Test visual acuity:**
   Snellen eye chart
   Near vision (patients older than 40 years or those having difficulty reading)
2. **Test visual fields:**
   Confrontation test
3. **Inspect extraocular muscle (EOM) function:**
   Corneal light reflex (Hirschberg test)
   Cover-uncover test
   Diagnostic positions test
4. **Inspect external eye structures:**
   General
   Eyebrows
   Eyelids and lashes
   Eyeball alignment
   Conjunctiva and sclera
   Lacrimal apparatus
5. **Inspect anterior eyeball structures:**
   Cornea and lens
   Iris and pupil
   Size, shape, and equality
   Pupillary light reflex
   Accommodation
6. **Inspect the ocular fundus:**
   Optic disc (colour, shape, margins, cup–disc ratio)
   Retinal vessels (number, colour, artery–vein ratio, calibre, arteriovenous crossings, tortuosity, pulsations)
   General background (colour, integrity)
   Macula
7. **Engage in teaching and health promotion**

ABNORMAL FINDINGS

TABLE 7.1   Aging Eye Changes

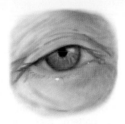

Relaxation of skin of upper eyelid

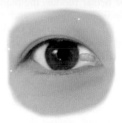

Pinguecula

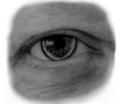

Arcus senilis

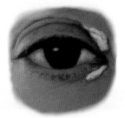

Xanthelasma

© Pat Thomas, 2010.

TABLE 7.2   Abnormalities in the Eyelids

Exophthalmos (Protruding Eyes)
Eyeballs are displaced forward, and palpebral fissures are widened. Note "lid lag"; the upper eyelid rests well above the limbus, and white sclera is visible. Acquired bilateral exophthalmos is associated with thyrotoxicosis.

Ptosis (Drooping Upper Eyelid)
Ptosis is caused by neuromuscular weakness (e.g., myasthenia gravis with bilateral fatigue as the day progresses), oculomotor cranial nerve III damage, or sympathetic nerve damage (e.g., Horner's syndrome).

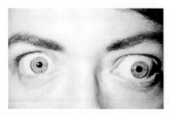

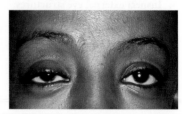

TABLE 7.2	Abnormalities in the Eyelids—cont'd

Ectropion

The lower lid is loose, rolls outward, and does not approximate to eyeball. Puncta cannot siphon tears effectively, so excess tearing results. Exposed palpebral conjunctiva increases risk for inflammation.

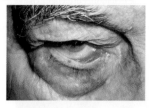

Entropion

The lower eyelid rolls inward because of spasm of eyelids or contraction of scar tissue. Constant rubbing of lashes may irritate cornea.

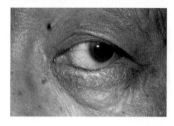

Chalazion

A beady nodule protruding on the eyelid, chalazion is an infection or retention cyst of a meibomian gland. It is a nontender, firm, discrete swelling with freely movable skin overlying the nodule. If it becomes inflamed, it points inside and not on the eyelid margin (in contrast with a stye).

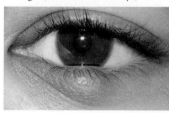

Hordeolum (Stye)

Hordeolum is a localized staphylococcal infection of the hair follicles at the eyelid margin. It is painful, red, and swollen; a pustule at the eyelid margin.

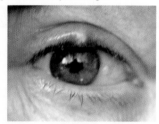

Continued

TABLE 7.2	Abnormalities in the Eyelids—cont'd

Basal Cell Carcinoma

Carcinoma is rare, but it occurs most often on the lower eyelid and medial canthus. It looks like a papule with an ulcerated centre. The edges are rolled out and pearly.

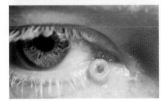

Conjunctivitis

Infection of the conjunctiva ("pink eye") shows red, beefy-looking vessels at the periphery, but usually looks clearer around the iris. This is a common symptom of bacterial or viral infection, allergy, or chemical irritation. Purulent discharge accompanies bacterial infection. Often accompanies an upper respiratory infection.

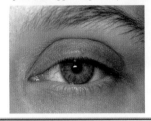

See Illustration Credits for source information.

TABLE 7.3	Abnormalities in the Pupil

Unequal Pupil Size: Anisocoria

Although anisocoria exists normally in 5% of the population, consider central nervous system disease.

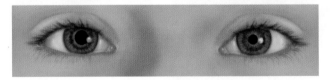

Monocular Blindness

When light is directed to the blind eye (in this illustration, the right eye), no response occurs in either eye. When light is directed to normal (left) eye, both pupils constrict (direct and consensual response to light) as long as the oculomotor nerve is intact.

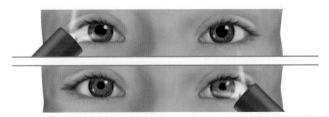

TABLE 7.3	Abnormalities in the Pupil—cont'd

Constricted and Fixed Pupils: Miosis

Miosis occurs with the use of pilocarpine drops for glaucoma treatment, the use of narcotics, with iritis, and with damage of the pons in the brain.

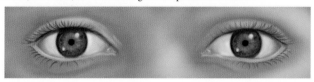

Dilated and Fixed Pupils: Mydriasis

Enlarged pupils occur with stimulation of the sympathetic nervous system, as a reaction to sympathomimetic drugs, with use of dilating drops, as a result of acute glaucoma, and with past or recent trauma. Enlarged pupils also indicate central nervous system injury, circulatory arrest, or deep anaesthesia.

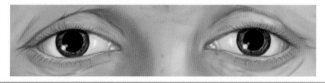

See Illustration Credits for source information.

··· ·········· ·······, ·· ········ ·········

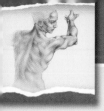

Ears

STRUCTURE AND FUNCTION

The ear is the sensory organ for hearing and maintaining equilibrium. The external ear is called the **auricle,** or **pinna,** and consists of movable cartilage and skin (Fig. 8.1).

The external ear funnels sound waves into its opening, the **external auditory canal.** The canal is a cul-de-sac, 2.5 to 3 cm long in the adult, and has a slight S-shaped curve (Fig. 8.2).

The middle ear is a tiny, air-filled cavity inside the temporal bone containing the tiny ear bones, or auditory ossicles: the **malleus, incus,** and **stapes.**

The inner ear is embedded in bone. It contains the **bony labyrinth,** which holds the sensory organs for equilibrium and hearing.

The **tympanic membrane,** or **eardrum,** separates the external ear and middle ear (Fig. 8.3). It is a translucent, pearly grey membrane in which a prominent cone of light in the anteroinferior quadrant is the reflection of the otoscope light.

The parts of the malleus show through the translucent eardrum; these are the **umbo,** the **manubrium** (handle), and the **short process.**

SOCIAL DETERMINANTS OF HEALTH CONSIDERATIONS

Cerumen is genetically determined and comes in two major types: (a) dry

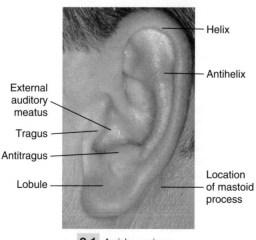

External auditory meatus

Tragus

Antitragus

Lobule

Helix

Antihelix

Location of mastoid process

8.1 Auricle, or pinna.

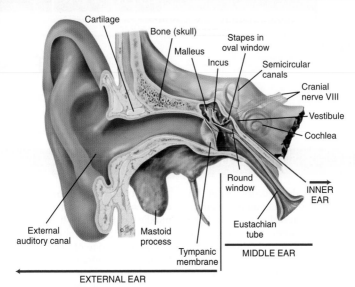

Cartilage
Bone (skull)
Malleus
Stapes in
oval window
Incus
Semicircular
canals
Cranial
nerve VIII
Vestibule
Cochlea
External
auditory canal
Mastoid
process
Round
window
INNER
EAR
Eustachian
tube
Tympanic
membrane
MIDDLE EAR
EXTERNAL EAR

8.2 Internal ear structures. *(© Pat Thomas, 2010.)*

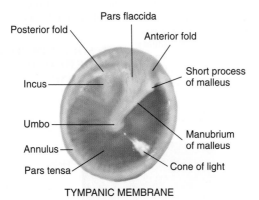

Pars flaccida
Posterior fold
Anterior fold
Short process
of malleus
Incus
Umbo
Manubrium
of malleus
Annulus
Pars tensa
Cone of light

TYMPANIC MEMBRANE

8.3 Tympanic membrane (eardrum).

cerumen, which is grey, flaky, and frequently forms a thin mass in the ear canal; and (b) wet cerumen, which is honey brown to dark brown and moist. Among individuals of Asian or Indigenous descent, frequency of dry cerumen exceeds 80%, whereas among individuals of African or Euro-Canadian descent, the frequency of wet cerumen exceeds 97%.

Otitis media (middle ear infection) is one of the most common illnesses in children. Besides the anatomy of the infant eustachian tube, the following risk factors predispose children to acute otitis media: absence of breastfeeding in the first 3 months of age, exposure to **secondhand tobacco smoke,** daycare attendance, male sex, pacifier use, low birth weight, low socioeconomic status, and bottle feeding in the supine position.

SUBJECTIVE DATA

1. Earache
2. Infections
3. Discharge
4. Hearing loss
5. Environmental noise

6. Tinnitus
7. Vertigo
8. Self-care behaviours (hearing last checked, method of cleaning ears)

OBJECTIVE DATA

PREPARATION

An adult should be sitting up straight with his or her head at your eye level.

EQUIPMENT NEEDED

Otoscope with bright light (fresh batteries give off white—not yellow— light)
Pneumatic bulb attachment, sometimes used with infants or young children

Normal Range of Findings	Abnormal Findings
Inspect and Palpate the External Ear	
Size and Shape	
The ears are of equal size bilaterally with no swelling or thickening.	*Microtia:* ears smaller than 4 cm vertically. *Macrotia:* ears larger than 10 cm vertically. Edema.
Skin Condition	
The skin is intact, with no lumps or lesions. **Darwin's tubercle,** a small painless nodule at the helix, is sometimes present. This is a congenital variation and is not significant.	Reddened, excessively warm skin: indicates inflammation. Crusts and scaling: occur with otitis externa, eczema, contact dermatitis, and seborrhea. Enlarged, tender lymph nodes in the region: indicate inflammation of the pinna or mastoid process. Red-blue discoloration: indicates frostbite. Tophi, sebaceous crust, chondrodermatitis, keloid, carcinoma. (See Table 16.2, p. 370, in Jarvis: *Physical Examination and Health Assessment,* 3rd Canadian edition.)

Continued

Normal Range of Findings	Abnormal Findings

Tenderness

Move the pinna and push on the tragus. They should feel firm, and movement should produce no pain. Palpating the mastoid process should also be painless.

Pain with movement: occurs with otitis externa and furuncle.

Pain at the mastoid process: may indicate mastoiditis or lymphadenitis of the posterior auricular node.

The External Auditory Meatus

There should be no swelling, redness, or discharge present.

Atresia: absence or closure of the ear canal.

Sticky yellow discharge: accompanies otitis externa, or it may indicate otitis media if the eardrum has ruptured.

Some cerumen is usually present. The colour varies from grey-yellow to light brown and black, and the texture varies from moist and waxy to dry and desiccated.

Impacted cerumen is a common cause of conductive hearing loss.

Inspect With the Otoscope

Choose the largest speculum that will fit comfortably in the ear canal. Tilt the patient's head slightly away from you toward the opposite shoulder. This method brings the obliquely sloping eardrum into better view.

Pull the pinna up and back on adults or older children (Fig. 8.4); this helps straighten the S-shaped curve of the canal. (Pull the pinna down on infants and children younger than 3 years of age.)

Hold the otoscope upside down along your fingers, and have the dorsa (back) of that hand along the patient's cheek braced to steady the otoscope (see Fig. 8.4).

Normal Range of Findings	Abnormal Findings

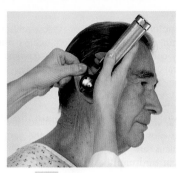

8.4   Using an otoscope.

The External Canal

Note any redness and swelling, lesions, foreign bodies, or discharge. If any discharge is present, note the colour and odour. (Also, clean any discharge off the speculum before examining the other ear, to avoid contamination with possibly infectious material.) For a patient with a hearing aid, note any irritation on the canal wall from poorly fitting ear moulds.

Redness and swelling occur with otitis externa; the canal may be completely closed with swelling.

Purulent otorrhea suggests otitis externa or otitis media if the eardrum has ruptured.

Frank blood or clear, watery drainage (cerebrospinal fluid) after trauma suggests basal skull fracture and warrants immediate referral. Cerebrospinal fluid feels oily and tests positive for glucose.

Foreign body, polyp, furuncle, and exostosis. (See Table 16.4, p. 373, in Jarvis: *Physical Examination and Health Assessment,* 3rd Canadian edition.)

Continued

Normal Range of Findings	Abnormal Findings

The Tympanic Membrane

Colour and Characteristics. The normal eardrum is shiny and translucent, with pearly-grey coloration (see Fig. 8.3). The cone-shaped light reflex is prominent in the anteroinferior quadrant (at the 5:00 position in the right eardrum and the 7:00 position in the left eardrum). This light reflex is the reflection of your otoscope light. Sections of the malleus are visible through the translucent eardrum: the umbo, manubrium, and short process. (Infrequently, the incus behind the eardrum shows as a whitish haze in the upper posterior area.) At the periphery, the annulus looks whiter and denser.

Yellow-amber eardrum discoloration: occurs with otitis media with effusion (serous).

Redness: occurs with acute otitis media.

Absence or distortion of landmarks.

Air/fluid level or air bubbles behind the eardrum: indicate otitis media with effusion (see Table 8.1).

Position. The eardrum is flat and slightly pulled in at the centre.

Retracted eardrum resulting from vacuum in middle ear with obstructed eustachian tube.

Bulging eardrum from increased pressure in otitis media.

Eardrum hypomobility is an early sign of otitis media (see Table 8.1).

Integrity of Membrane. The normal tympanic membrane is intact. Some adults may show scarring, which is a dense white patch on the drum. This is a sequela of repeated ear infections.

Perforation: a dark oval area or a larger opening on the eardrum (see Table 8.1).

Normal Range of Findings	Abnormal Findings

Test Hearing Acuity

Whispered Voice Test

Stand arm's length (half a meter, or 2 feet) behind the person. Test one ear at a time while masking hearing in the other ear to prevent sound transmission around the head. This is done by placing one finger on the tragus and pushing it in and out of the auditory meatus. Move your head to about half a meter (2 feet) from the person's ear. Exhale fully and slowly whisper a set of 3 random numbers and letters, such as "5, B, 6." Normally the person repeats each number/letter correctly after you say it. If the response is not correct, repeat the whispered test using a different combination of 3 numbers and letters. A passing score is correct repetition of at least 3 of a possible 6 numbers/letters (Walling & Dickson, 2012).

Inability to hear whispered words (a whisper is a high-frequency sound and is used to detect high-tone loss).

Tuning Fork Tests

Tuning fork tests measure hearing by air conduction or bone conduction in which the sound vibrates through the cranial bones to the inner ear. The air conduction route through the ear canal and middle ear is usually the more sensitive route. Traditionally, these tests have been taught for physical examination, but evidence shows that both the Weber and Rinne tuning fork tests do not yield precise or reliable data. Thus, these tests should not be used for general screening.

 DEVELOPMENTAL CONSIDERATIONS

Infants and Young Children

The top of the pinna should be horizontally aligned with the corner of the eye to the occiput, and the ear should be positioned within 10 degrees of vertical.

Low-set ears or deviation in alignment may indicate intellectual disability or a genitourinary malformation.

Continued

Normal Range of Findings	Abnormal Findings

Remember to pull the pinna straight down on an infant or child younger than 3 years. This method will help match the slope of the ear canal.

When examining an infant or young child, a pneumatic bulb attachment on the otoscope enables you to direct a light puff of air toward the drum to assess **vibratility** (Fig. 8.5). For a secure seal, choose the largest speculum that will fit the ear canal without causing pain. A rubber tip on the end of the speculum gives a better seal. Give a small pump to the bulb (positive pressure), then release the bulb (negative pressure). Normally, the tympanic membrane moves inward with a slight puff and outward with a slight release. Normally, the eardrum is intact. In a child being treated for chronic otitis media, you may note the presence of a tympanostomy tube in the central part of the eardrum. This is inserted surgically to equalize pressure and drain secretions. It is common, although not normal, to note a foreign body in a child's ear canal, such as a small stone or a bead.

An abnormal response is no movement of the eardrum. Eardrum hypomobility indicates effusion or a high vacuum in the middle ear. For the newborn's first 6 weeks, eardrum immobility is the best indicator of middle ear infection.

Chronic otitis media relieved by tympanostomy tubes. (See Table 16.4, p. 373, in Jarvis: *Physical Examination and Health Assessment,* 3rd Canadian edition.)

Foreign body. (See Table 16.4, p. 373, in Jarvis: *Physical Examination and Health Assessment,* 3rd Canadian edition.)

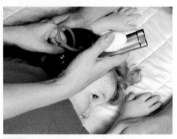

8.5 Using an otoscope with pneumatic bulb attachment.

Normal Range of Findings	Abnormal Findings

Older Adults

Earlobes may be pendulous with linear wrinkling because of loss of elasticity of the pinna. Coarse, wiry hairs may be present at the opening of the ear canal. During otoscopy, the drum may normally be whiter in colour, more opaque, and duller than in the younger adult. It also may look thickened.

High-tone frequency hearing loss is apparent for those affected with **presbycusis,** the hearing loss that occurs with aging. Note any difficulty hearing in the whispered voice test and difficulty hearing consonants during conversational speech.

For more information on assessment of the ears and hearing, see Chapter 16, page 358, in Jarvis: *Physical Examination and Health Assessment,* 3rd Canadian edition.

Summary Checklist: Ear Examination

1. **Inspect external ear:**
   Size and shape of pinna
   Position and alignment on head
   Skin condition: colour, lumps, lesions
   Movement of pinna and tragus (check for tenderness)
   External auditory meatus: size, swelling, redness, discharge, cerumen, lesions, foreign bodies
2. **Otoscopic examination:**
   External canal
   Cerumen, discharge, foreign bodies, lesions
   Redness or swelling of canal wall
3. **Inspect eardrum:**
   Colour and characteristics
   Position (flat, bulging, retracted)
   Integrity of membrane (no perforations)
4. **Test hearing acuity:**
   Behavioural response to conversational speech
   Voice test
5. **Engage in teaching and health promotion**

ABNORMAL FINDINGS

TABLE 8.1	Abnormalities of the Ear Canal or Tympanic Membrane

Excessive Cerumen

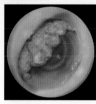

Excessive cerumen is produced or is impacted because of a narrow tortuous canal or poor cleaning method. It may appear as a round ball partially obscuring the eardrum or totally occluding the canal. Even when the canal is 90–95% blocked, hearing stays normal; when the last 5–10% is totally occluded (when cerumen expands after swimming or showering), the patient has the sensation of ear fullness and sudden hearing loss.

Otitis Externa (Swimmer's Ear)

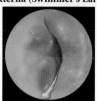

Severe swelling of canal; inflammation; tenderness. In this illustration, canal lumen is narrowed to one-fourth of normal size. An infection of the outer ear, with severe painful movement of pinna and tragus, redness and swelling of pinna and canal, scanty purulent discharge, scaling, itching, fever, and enlarged tender regional lymph nodes. Hearing is normal or slightly diminished. More common in hot, humid weather. Swimming causes canal to become waterlogged and swell; skinfolds are set up for infection.

Retracted Eardrum

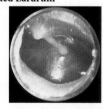

Landmarks look more prominent and well defined. Malleus handle looks shorter and more horizontal than normal. Short process is very prominent. Light reflex is absent or distorted. The eardrum is dull and lustreless and does not move. These signs indicate negative pressure and middle ear vacuum caused by obstruction of eustachian tube and serous otitis media.

Acute (Purulent) Otitis Media

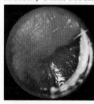

This results when the middle ear fluid is infected. Absence of light reflex as a result of increasing middle ear pressure is an early sign. Redness and bulging are first noted in superior part of eardrum (pars flaccida; *left photo*), along with earache and fever. Then fiery red and bulging of entire eardrum *(right photo)*, deep throbbing pain, fever, and transient hearing loss occur. Pneumatic otoscopy reveals eardrum hypomobility.

TABLE 8.1	Abnormalities of the Ear Canal or Tympanic Membrane—cont'd

Otitis Media With Effusion

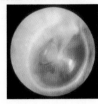

Perforation

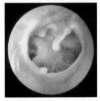

An amber-yellow eardrum, an air/fluid level with fine black dividing line, or air bubbles visible behind eardrum. Symptoms are sensation of fullness, transient hearing loss, popping sound with swallowing. Also called *serous otitis media* and *glue ear*.

Eardrum rupture from increased pressure or from trauma (e.g., a slap on the ear). Usually, the perforation appears as a round or oval darkened area on the eardrum, but in this photo the perforation is very large. *Central* perforations occur in the pars tensa, and *marginal* perforations occur at the annulus.

See Illustration Credits for source information.

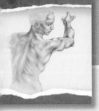

CHAPTER 9

Nose, Mouth, and Throat

STRUCTURE AND FUNCTION

The **nose** is the first segment of the respiratory system. It warms, moistens, and filters the inhaled air, and it is the sensory organ for smell.

The oval openings at the base of the nose are the *nares* (Fig. 9.1). The *columella* divides the two nares and is continuous inside with the nasal septum.

Inside, the **nasal cavity** is large and extends back over the roof of the mouth (Fig. 9.2). Nasal mucosa appears redder than oral mucosa because of the rich blood supply present to warm the inhaled air.

The lateral walls of each nasal cavity contain three parallel bony projections: the superior, middle, and inferior **turbinates.** They increase the surface area so that more blood vessels and mucous membranes are available to warm, humidify, and filter the inhaled air.

The **mouth** is the first segment of the digestive system and an airway for the respiratory system (Fig. 9.3). It contains the teeth and gums, tongue, and salivary glands. The anterior **hard palate** is made up of bone and is a whitish colour; the more posterior **soft palate** is an arch of muscle that is pinker and mobile.

The **throat,** or **pharynx,** is the area behind the mouth and nose. The **oropharynx** is separated from the mouth by two folds of tissue, the anterior tonsillar pillars, one on each side. Behind the folds are the **tonsils,** each a mass of lymphoid tissue. The **nasopharynx** is continuous with the oropharynx, although it is above the oropharynx and behind the

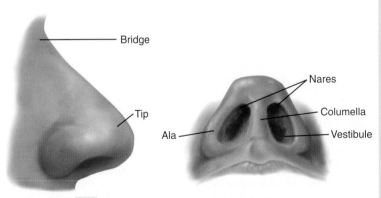

Bridge

Tip

Ala

Nares

Columella

Vestibule

9.1 External nasal structures. *(© Pat Thomas, 2006.)*

95

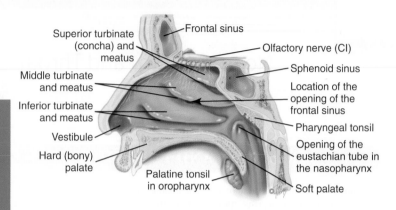

RIGHT LATERAL WALL—NASAL CAVITY

9.2 Internal nasal structures. *(© Pat Thomas, 2006.)*

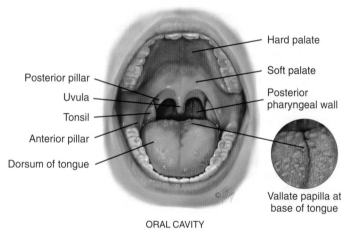

ORAL CAVITY

9.3 Mouth structures. *(© Pat Thomas, 2010.)*

nasal cavity. The pharyngeal tonsils (adenoids) and the eustachian tube openings are located here.

CULTURAL AND SOCIAL DETERMINANTS OF HEALTH CONSIDERATIONS

The incidence of **cleft palate** is the same across ethnic groups, but Indigenous peoples have a higher occurrence of **cleft lip** and combined cleft lip/cleft palate. Torus palatinus, a bony ridge running down the middle of the hard palate, is also more common in Indigenous people and people of Asian descent. **Leukoedema,** a greyish-white benign lesion occurring on the buccal mucosa, may be present in people of African descent. Oral hyperpigmentation also varies according to ethnocultural groups. Usually absent at birth, hyperpigmentation increases with age; it is more common among people of African descent and is believed to be caused by a lifetime accumulation of post-inflammatory oral changes.

Indigenous peoples, recent refugees and immigrants, individuals from lower socioeconomic groups, people with disabilities, and Canadians living in rural or remote areas are less likely to have access to regular, comprehensive dental care, resulting in a greater prevalence of edentulism, periodontal disease, dental pain, and chewing difficulties among these populations (Canadian Academy of Health Sciences, 2014).

Body piercing is the establishment of an unnatural tract through tissue that is held open by artificial means. The nose is the most common site for oral piercing, followed by the mouth, and tongue. Infection is the most frequent complication of piercings, with infection rates ranging from 9% to 35% (Bellaud et al., 2017). As a pierced site provides a route of entry for microorganisms, a localized or systemic infection may occur. Additional oral complications include abnormal tooth wear, tooth chipping/cracking, tooth loss, and periodontal disease (Duval Smith, 2016).

SUBJECTIVE DATA

Nose
1. Discharge
2. Frequent colds (upper respiratory infections)
3. Sinus pain
4. Trauma
5. Epistaxis (nosebleeds)
6. Allergies
7. Altered smell

Mouth and Throat
1. Sores or lesions
2. Sore throat

3. Bleeding gums
4. Toothache
5. Sugar consumption
6. Bruxism (teeth grinding)
7. Hoarseness
8. Dysphagia
9. Altered taste
10. Tobacco consumption
11. Alcohol consumption
12. Sleep apnea
13. Self-care behaviours (oral care pattern, dentures, or appliances)

OBJECTIVE DATA

PREPARATION
Position the patient sitting up straight with his or her head at your eye level. If the patient wears dentures, offer a paper towel and ask the patient to remove them.*

EQUIPMENT NEEDED
Otoscope with short, wide-tipped nasal speculum attachment
Penlight
Two tongue blades
Cotton gauze pad (10 × 10 cm)
Gloves*
Occasionally: long-stem light attachment for otoscope

*Always wear gloves to examine mucous membranes, in accordance with routine practices to prevent spread of communicable diseases.

Normal Range of Findings	Abnormal Findings

Inspect and Palpate the Nose

External Nose

Normally, the nose is midline, symmetrical, and in proportion to other facial features. Inspect for any deformity, asymmetry, inflammation, or skin lesions.

Test the patency of the nostrils by pushing one nasal wing shut with your finger while asking the patient to sniff inward through the other naris, and repeat on the other side. This reveals any obstruction, which can later be explored using the nasal speculum.

Absence of sniff indicates obstruction (e.g., common cold, nasal polyps, and rhinitis).

Nasal Cavity

Attach the short, wide-tipped speculum to the otoscope head and insert into the nasal vestibule, avoiding pressure on the nasal septum (Fig. 9.4).

Inspect the nasal mucosa, noting its normal red colour and smooth moist surface (Fig. 9.5). Note any swelling, discharge, bleeding, or foreign body (see Table 9.1).

Nasal mucosa is swollen and bright red with rhinitis and upper respiratory infection.

Discharge is common with rhinitis and sinusitis, varying from watery and copious to thick, purulent, and green-yellow.

With chronic allergy, mucosa looks swollen, boggy, pale, and grey.

For more information on abnormalities of the nose, see Table 17.1, p. 406, in Jarvis: *Physical Examination and Health Assessment,* 3rd Canadian edition.

Normal Range of Findings	Abnormal Findings

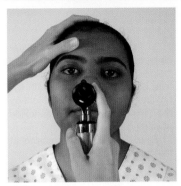

9.4   Inserting the otoscope into the nasal vestibule.

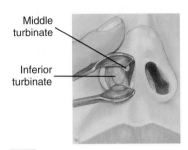

Middle turbinate

Inferior turbinate

9.5   Viewing the naris through nasal speculum.

Observe the nasal septum for deviation, perforation, or bleeding. A deviated septum is common and is only significant if airflow is obstructed.

Inspect the turbinates, the bony ridges curving down from the lateral walls. The superior turbinate is not in your view, but middle and inferior turbinates appear the same light red colour as the nasal mucosa. Note any swelling, but do not try to push the speculum past it. Turbinates are quite vascular and tender if touched.

Note any polyps, benign growths that accompany chronic allergy, and distinguish them from normal turbinates.

A deviated septum looks like a hump or shelf in one nasal cavity.

Perforation is visible as a spot of light from the penlight shining in other naris and occurs with cocaine use.

Epistaxis commonly comes from the anterior septum.

Polyps are smooth, pale grey, avascular, mobile, and nontender.

Palpate the Sinus Areas

Using your thumbs, press over the frontal sinuses below the eyebrows and over the maxillary sinuses below the cheekbones. Take care not to palpate below the bony orbitals (eye sockets) to avoid pressing the eyeballs. The patient should feel firm pressure but no pain.

Sinus areas are tender to palpation in patients with chronic allergies and acute infection (sinusitis).

Continued

Normal Range of Findings	Abnormal Findings

Inspect the Mouth

Lips

Inspect the lips for colour, moisture, cracking, or lesions. Retract lips and note their inner surface. Individuals with darker complexions may normally have bluish lips and a dark line on the gingival margin.

In light-skinned people, whiteness around the lips (circumoral pallor) occurs with shock and anemia; bluish lips (cyanosis) with hypoxemia and chilling; and cherry red lips with carbon monoxide poisoning.

Cheilitis (perlèche): cracking at the corners.

Herpes simplex, other lesions (see Table 9.2).

Teeth and Gums

Teeth normally appear white, straight, evenly spaced, clean, and free of debris or decay. Note any diseased, absent, loose, or abnormally positioned teeth.

Discoloured teeth appear brown with excessive fluoride use, and yellow with tobacco use.

Periodontal disease is linked to cardiovascular disease, diabetes, pulmonary infections, kidney disease, and osteoporosis.

Grinding down of tooth surface.

Plaque: soft debris.

Caries: decay.

Enamel erosion: eating disorder.

Malocclusion: protrusion of upper or lower incisors.

Ask the patient to bite as if chewing something, and note alignment of upper and lower jaw. Normal occlusion in the back is the upper teeth resting directly on the lower teeth; in the front, the upper incisors slightly override the lower incisors.

Normally, the gums look pink or coral with a stippled (dotted) surface. The gum margins are tight and well-defined. Check for swelling, retraction of gingival margins, and spongy, bleeding, or discoloured gums. Individuals with darker complexions may normally have a dark melanotic line along the gingival margin.

Gingival hyperplasia, crevices between teeth and gums, pockets of debris.

Gums bleed with slight pressure, indicating gingivitis.

Dark line on gingival margins occurs with lead and bismuth poisoning.

Normal Range of Findings	Abnormal Findings

Tongue

The tongue colour is pink and even. The dorsal surface is normally roughened from the papillae. A thin white coating may be present. Ask the patient to touch the tongue to the roof of the mouth. Its ventral surface looks smooth, glistening, and shows veins. Saliva is present.

Beefy red, swollen tongue.

Smooth glossy areas. (See Table 17.5, p. 414, in Jarvis: *Physical Examination and Health Assessment,* 3rd Canadian edition.)

Enlarged tongue (macroglossia) occurs with allergic and anaphylactic reactions, hypothyroidism, and acromegaly.

Dry mouth occurs with dehydration, fever; tongue has deep vertical fissures.

Saliva is decreased while the patient is taking anticholinergic and other medications. Excessive saliva and drooling occur with gingivostomatitis and neurological dysfunction.

With a glove on, carefully inspect the tongue and the entire U-shaped area under the tongue behind the teeth. Note any white patches, nodules, or ulcerations. If lesions are present, or with any patient older than 50 years, or with a positive history of smoking or alcohol use, use your gloved hand to palpate the area. Notice any firmness or induration.

Any lesion or ulcer persisting for more than 2 weeks must be investigated.

A hardened area may be a mass or lymphadenopathy and must be investigated.

Buccal Mucosa

The buccal mucosa looks pink, smooth, and moist, although patchy hyperpigmentation is common and normal in dark-skinned people.

Dappled brown patches are present with Addison's disease (chronic adrenal insufficiency).

Continued

Normal Range of Findings	Abnormal Findings
Stensen's duct, the opening of the parotid salivary gland, looks like a small dimple opposite the upper second molar. You may also see a raised occlusion line on the buccal mucosa parallel with the level at which the teeth meet; this is caused by the teeth closing against the cheek.	The orifice of Stensen's duct becomes red with mumps. **Koplik's spots:** small blue-white spots that are an early prodromal (early warning) sign of measles. **Leukoplakia,** a chalky white raised patch, is abnormal. (See Table 17.4, p. 412, in Jarvis: *Physical Examination and Health Assessment,* 3rd Canadian edition.) *Candida* infection will usually rub off, leaving a clear or raw denuded surface.
Fordyce's granules are small, isolated white or yellow papules on the mucosa of the cheek, tongue, and lips. These little sebaceous cysts are painless and not significant.	
Palate	
The more anterior hard palate is white with irregular transverse rugae. The posterior soft palate is pinker, smooth, and upwardly movable. A normal variation is a **torus palatinus,** a nodular bony ridge down the middle of the hard palate (see Table 9.2).	The hard palate appears yellow with jaundice. In dark-skinned people with jaundice, it may look yellow, muddy yellow, or green-brown. **Oral Kaposi's sarcoma** is a bruiselike, dark red or violet, confluent macular lesion, usually on the hard palate. It is the most common early lesion in people with acquired immune deficiency syndrome (AIDS).
Ask the patient to say "ahhh," and note the soft palate and uvula rise in the midline. This tests one function of cranial nerve X, the vagus nerve.	A **bifid uvula** appears as if split in two; it is more common in Indigenous people. (See Table 17.6, p. 415, in Jarvis: *Physical Examination and Health Assessment,* 3rd Canadian edition.)
Notice any breath odour (*halitosis*). This is common and usually has a local cause, such as poor oral hygiene, consumption of odoriferous foods, alcohol consumption, heavy smoking, or dental infection. Occasionally, it indicates systemic disease.	Diabetic ketoacidosis produces a sweet, fruity breath odour; this acetone smell also occurs in children with malnutrition or dehydration. Other breath odours include ammonia, which occurs with uremia; a musty odour, with liver disease; a foul, fetid odour, with dental or respiratory infections; and an alcohol odour, with alcohol or chemical ingestion.

Normal Range of Findings	Abnormal Findings

Inspect the Throat

The **tonsils** are the same pink as the oral mucosa, and their surface is peppered with indentations, or crypts. In some people, the crypts collect small plugs of whitish cellular debris. This does not indicate infection. Tonsils are graded in size as follows:

1+: Visible
2+: Halfway between tonsillar pillars and uvula
3+: Touching the uvula
4+: Touching each other

You may normally see grade 1+ or grade 2+ tonsils in healthy people, especially in children.

Depress the tongue with a tongue blade. Scan the posterior wall for colour, exudate, and lesions. When finished, discard the tongue blade.

Touching the posterior wall with the tongue blade elicits the gag reflex. This tests cranial nerves IX and X, the glossopharyngeal and vagus nerves.

Test cranial nerve XII, the hypoglossal nerve, by asking the patient to stick out the tongue. It should protrude in the midline. Children enjoy this request. Note any tremor, loss of movement, or deviation to the side.

✦ **DEVELOPMENTAL CONSIDERATIONS**

Infants and Children

Nose. The newborn may have milia across the nose. The nasal bridge may be flat in Indigenous children and in children of Asian or African descent. There should be no nasal flaring or narrowing with breathing.

With an acute infection, tonsils are bright red, swollen, and may have exudates or large white spots.

A white membrane covering the tonsils may accompany infectious mononucleosis, leukemia, and diphtheria.

Tonsils are enlarged to 2+, 3+, or 4+ with an acute infection.

You can help the patient with an easily triggered gag reflex by offering to let them depress their tongue with the tongue blade. (Some people can lower their own tongue, so the tongue blade is not needed.) If the tongue blade does not help to visualize the posterior wall, the client should be asked to say "ahhh" to help.

With damage to cranial nerve XII, the tongue deviates *toward* the paralyzed side. A fine tremor of the tongue occurs with hyperthyroidism; a coarse tremor, with cerebral palsy, and alcoholism.

Nasal flaring in the infant indicates respiratory distress.

Many children with chronic allergy have a transverse ridge across the nose, caused by wiping the nose upward with the palm.

Nasal narrowing on inhalation is seen with chronic nasal obstruction and mouth breathing.

Continued

Normal Range of Findings	Abnormal Findings

Mouth and Throat. Note the number of teeth and whether this number is appropriate for the child's age. Also note patterns of eruption, position, condition, and hygiene. Use this guide for children younger than 2 years: the child's age in months minus the number 6 should equal the expected number of deciduous teeth. Normally, all 20 deciduous teeth are in by 2½ years of age.

Note any bruising or laceration on buccal mucosa or gums of infant or young child.

No teeth by age 1 year is abnormal.

Discoloured teeth appear yellow or yellow-brown with infants taking tetracycline or whose mothers took the drug during the last trimester; appear green or black with excessive iron ingestion, although this reverses when the iron is stopped.

Nursing bottle caries are brown discolourations on upper front teeth from taking a bottle of milk, juice, or sweetened drink into bed.

Trauma may indicate child abuse resulting from forced feeding of bottle or spoon.

Pregnant Women

Gum hypertrophy (surface looks smooth and stippling disappears) may occur normally at puberty or during pregnancy (pregnancy gingivitis). Gums may bleed as a result of increased hormone production, which causes increased vascularity and fragility. Proper oral hygiene and healthy food choices help prevent pregnancy gingivitis.

Older Adults

The nose may appear more prominent on the face from a loss of subcutaneous fat.

In the edentulous patient, the mouth and lips fold in, giving a "purse-string" appearance. The teeth may look slightly yellowed, though the colour is uniform. The teeth may look longer as the gum margins recede. Tooth surfaces look worn down or abraded. Old dental work deteriorates, especially at the gum margins. The teeth loosen with bone resorption and may move with palpation. The tongue looks smoother because of papillary atrophy. The older adult's buccal mucosa is thinned and may look shinier, as though it were varnished.

Summary Checklist: Nose, Mouth, and Throat Examination

Nose
1. **Inspect external nose:**
   Symmetry
   Any deformity
   Lesions
2. **Palpate to test patency of each nostril**
3. **Inspect nasal cavity using nasal speculum:**
   Nasal mucosa for colour and integrity
   Septum for deviation, perforation, or bleeding
   Turbinates for colour, any exudate, swelling, or polyps
4. **Palpate the sinus areas: note any tenderness**

Mouth and Throat
1. **Inspect using penlight:**
   Lips, teeth and gums, tongue, buccal mucosa
   Colour, intactness of structures, any lesions
   Palate and uvula
   Integrity and mobility as patient phonates
   Grade tonsils
   Pharyngeal wall for colour, any exudate, or lesions
2. **Palpate:**
   When indicated in adults, palpate mouth bimanually.
   With the neonate, palpate for integrity of the palate and to assess sucking reflex

ABNORMAL FINDINGS

TABLE 9.1	Abnormalities of the Nose

Foreign Body

Children are particularly apt to put an object up the nose (here, yellow plastic foam), which leads to unilateral mucopurulent drainage and foul odour. Because some risk for aspiration exists, removal should be prompt.

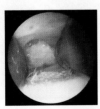

Perforated Septum

A hole in the septum, usually in the cartilaginous part, may be caused by snorting cocaine, chronic infection, trauma from continual picking of crusts, or nasal surgery. It is seen directly, or as a spot of light when the penlight is directed into the other naris.

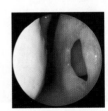

Continued

TABLE 9.1	Abnormalities of the Nose—cont'd

Acute Rhinitis

The first sign is a clear, watery discharge, rhinorrhea, which later becomes purulent. This is accompanied by sneezing and swollen mucosa, which causes nasal obstruction. Turbinates are dark red and swollen.

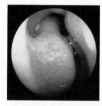

Allergic Rhinitis

Rhinorrhea, itching of nose and eyes, lacrimation, nasal congestion, and sneezing are present. Note serous edema and swelling of turbinates to fill the air space. Turbinates are usually pale (although they may appear violet), and their surface looks smooth and glistening. May be seasonal or perennial, depending on allergen. Affected individual often has a strong family history of seasonal allergies.

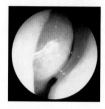

See Illustration Credits for source information.

TABLE 9.2	Abnormalities of the Mouth and Throat

Angular Cheilitis (Stomatitis, Perlèche)

Erythema, scaling, and shallow and painful fissures at the corners of the mouth occur with excess salivation and *Candida* infection. Seen in edentulous patients and in those with poorly fitting dentures that cause folding in of corners of mouth.

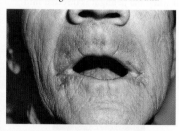

Gingivitis

Gum margins are red, swollen, and bleed easily. Inflammation is usually a result of poor dental hygiene or vitamin C deficiency. The condition may occur in pregnancy and puberty because of a change in hormonal balance.

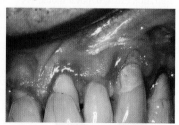

TABLE 9.2	Abnormalities of the Mouth and Throat—cont'd

Herpes Simplex I

"Cold sores" are groups of clear vesicles with a surrounding indurated erythematous base. These evolve into pustules, which rupture, weep, crust, and heal in 4–10 days. The most likely site is the lip–skin junction; infection often recurs in same site. Recurrent herpes infections may be precipitated by sunlight, fever, colds, and allergy. It is a very common lesion, affecting 50% of adults.

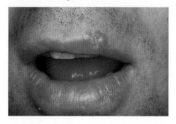

Aphthous Ulcers

Also called *canker sore;* are vesicles at first and then become small, round, "punched-out" ulcers with a white base surrounded by a red halo. They are quite painful and last for 1–2 weeks. The cause is unknown, although they are associated with stress, fatigue, and food allergy. They are common, affecting 20–60% of the population.

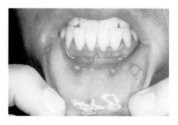

Torus Palatinus

A normal variation is a modular bony ridge down the middle of the hard palate (seen here using a mirror). This benign growth arises after puberty and is more common in Indigenous people or people of African or Asian descent.

Upper lip

Torus in upper hard palate

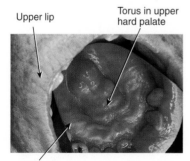

Mirror

Acute Tonsillitis and Pharyngitis

Bright red throat; swollen tonsils; white or yellow exudate on tonsils and pharynx; swollen uvula; and enlarged, tender anterior cervical and tonsillar nodes. Accompanied by severe sore throat, painful swallowing, and fever (temperature >38.3°C) of sudden onset.

Caution: Bacterial infection cannot be distinguished from viral infection on the basis of clinical data alone; all patients with sore throats need a throat culture. Bacterial pharyngitis caused by group A β-hemolytic *Streptococcus* species, if untreated, may lead to the complication of rheumatic fever. This is a serious, complex illness characterized by fever, malaise, swollen joints, rash, and scarring on the heart valves.

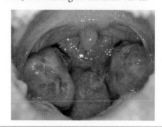

See Illustration Credits for source information.

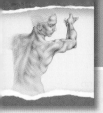

CHAPTER 10

Breasts and Regional Lymphatic System

STRUCTURE AND FUNCTION

The female **breasts** are accessory reproductive organs with a function of producing milk. The breasts lie anterior to the pectoralis major and serratus anterior muscles, between the second and sixth ribs (Fig. 10.1). The superior lateral corner of breast tissue, called the **axillary tail of Spence,** projects up and laterally into the axilla.

The breast may be viewed as four quadrants, with imaginary horizontal and vertical lines intersecting at the nipple. This makes a convenient map to describe clinical findings: upper outer, lower outer, lower inner, and upper inner quadrants.

Internally, the breast is composed of:

1. **Glandular tissue,** containing 15 to 20 lobes radiating from the nipple (Fig. 10.2). Each lobe empties into a **lactiferous** duct and these converge toward the nipple.

2. The suspensory ligaments, or **Cooper's ligaments,** are fibrous bands extending vertically from the surface to the chest wall muscles. They support the breast tissue.

3. The **adipose tissue.** These layers of subcutaneous and retromammary fat provide most of the bulk of the breast.

The breast has extensive lymphatic drainage (Fig. 10.3). Four groups of axillary nodes are present:

1. **Central axillary nodes,** high up in the middle of the axilla;

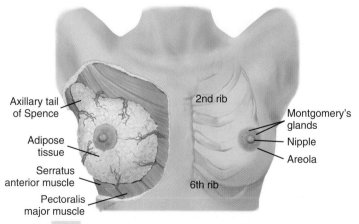

Axillary tail of Spence

Adipose tissue

Serratus anterior muscle

Pectoralis major muscle

2nd rib

Montgomery's glands

Nipple

Areola

6th rib

10.1 Surface anatomy of the breast. *(© Pat Thomas, 2010.)*

109

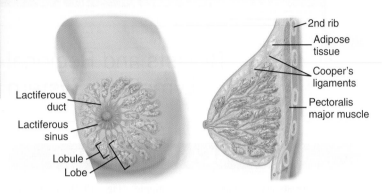

10.2 Internal anatomy: (a) glandular tissue, (b) fibrous tissue including suspensory ligaments, (c) adipose tissue. (© Pat Thomas, 2010.)

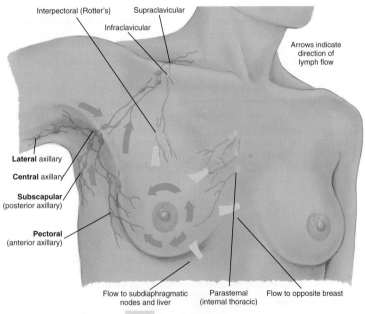

10.3 Lymphatic drainage.

2. **Pectoral** (anterior) nodes, along the lateral edge of the pectoralis major muscle;

3. **Subscapular** (posterior) nodes, along the lateral edge of the scapula; and

4. **Lateral** nodes, along the humerus, inside the upper arm.

From the central axillary nodes, drainage flows up to the infraclavicular and supraclavicular nodes.

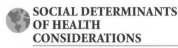

SOCIAL DETERMINANTS OF HEALTH CONSIDERATIONS

The lifetime risk for breast cancer in Canada is approximately 1 per 8, and 1 per 30 women may be expected to die from breast cancer (Canadian Cancer Statistics Advisory Committee, 2017). Incidence and mortality rates for breast cancer, and related risk factors, are heavily influenced by socioeconomic level, ethnocultural background, rural locations, and inequities in access to health services. For example, women of higher socioeconomic status have a slightly increased risk for breast cancer; researchers speculate that this may be related to an average older age at childbearing, having fewer children, or a greater likelihood of receiving postmenopausal hormone replacement therapy (Canadian Cancer Statistics Advisory Committee, 2017).

The growing obesity "epidemic" in Canada has important implications for breast cancer risk. Although obesity is an identified risk factor for breast cancer, and increased body mass index is associated with poor prognosis for breast cancer (Widschwendter et al., 2015), the relationship of breast cancer to dietary fat is not yet clear. It is clear, however, that the relationship between obesity, high-fat diets, and breast cancer has implications for Canadians who consume a "typical" high-fat North American–style diet and, in particular, for those who lack the socioeconomic resources to eat more nutritious foods. For example, Indigenous people living in far northern and remote communities may not be able to make more nutritious food choices because of both the high cost and the lack of availability of such foods in their communities.

SUBJECTIVE DATA

Breast
1. Pain
2. Lump
3. Discharge
4. Rash
5. Swelling
6. Trauma
7. History of breast disease

8. Surgery
9. Self-care behaviours
   • Perform breast self-examination
   • Last mammogram

Axilla
1. Tenderness, lump, or swelling
2. Rash

OBJECTIVE DATA

PREPARATION
The woman is sitting up, facing the examiner. Use a short gown, open at the back, and lift it up to the woman's shoulders during inspection. During palpation, the woman is supine; cover one breast with the gown while examining the other.

EQUIPMENT NEEDED
Small pillow
Ruler marked in centimetres

Normal Range of Findings	Abnormal Findings

Inspect the Breasts

General Appearance

Note symmetry of size and shape. It is common and normal to have a slight asymmetry in size; often the left breast is slightly larger than the right (Fig. 10.4).

A sudden increase in size of one breast signifies inflammation or new growth.

Skin

The skin is normally smooth and of even colour with no localized redness, bulging, dimpling, skin lesions, or focal vascular pattern. A fine blue vascular network is normal during pregnancy. Pale linear **striae**, or stretch marks, often follow pregnancy or periods of weight gain/loss.
Normally no edema is present.

Hyperpigmentation.
Redness and heat with inflammation.
Unilateral dilated superficial veins in a nonpregnant woman.

Edema exaggerates the hair follicles, giving a "pig skin" or "orange peel" look (also called *peau d'orange*).

Lymphatic Drainage Areas

The axillary and supraclavicular regions have no bulging, discolouration, or edema.

Nipple

The nipples should be symmetrical, on the same plane on the two breasts, and usually protrude, although some are flat and some are inverted. Distinguish a recently retracted nipple from one that has been inverted for many years or since puberty.

Deviation in pointing.
Recent nipple retraction signifies acquired disease. (See Table 18.3, p. 442, in Jarvis: *Physical Examination and Health Assessment,* 3rd Canadian edition.)

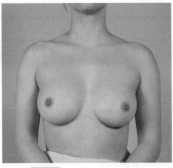

10.4 Breast appearance.

Normal Range of Findings	Abnormal Findings

Note any dry scaling, any fissure or ulceration, and bleeding or other discharge. Normally, there is none.

A supernumerary nipple is a normal and common variation. An extra nipple along the embryonic "milk line" on the thorax or abdomen is a congenital occurrence. Usually, it is 5 to 6 cm below the breast near the midline and looks like a mole, although a close look reveals a tiny nipple and areola. It is not significant.

Manoeuvres to Screen for Retraction

First ask the woman to lift her arms slowly over her head. Both breasts should move up symmetrically.

Next, ask her to put her hands on her hips and push, and then to push her two palms together. There will be a slight lifting of both breasts.

Inspect and Palpate the Axillae

Inspect the skin, noting any rash or infection. Lift the woman's arm and support it yourself so that her muscles are loose and relaxed. Reach your fingers high into the axilla and move them firmly down in four directions: (a) down the chest wall in a line from the middle of the axilla, (b) along the anterior border of the axilla, (c) along the posterior border, and (d) along the inner aspect of the upper arm.

Usually nodes are not palpable, although you may feel a small, soft, nontender node in the central group. Expect some tenderness when palpating high in the axilla. Note any enlarged and tender lymph nodes.

Any discharge must be explored, especially in the presence of a breast mass.

In rare cases, additional glandular tissue, called a *supernumerary breast,* is present.

Retraction signs result from fibrosis in the breast tissue, usually caused by growing neoplasms.

Note a lag in movement of one breast.

Note a dimpling or a pucker that indicates skin retraction. (See Table 18.3, p. 441, in Jarvis: *Physical Examination and Health Assessment,* 3rd Canadian edition.)

Nodes enlarge with any local infection of the breast, arm, or hand, and with breast cancer metastases.

Continued

Normal Range of Findings	Abnormal Findings

Palpate the Breasts

Help the woman into a supine position. Tuck a small pad under the side to be palpated and raise her arm over her head to flatten the breast tissue and displace it medially.

Use the pads of your first three fingers and make a gentle rotary motion on the breast. Vary your pressure so you are palpating light, medium, and deep tissues in each location. The vertical strip pattern (Fig. 10.5, *A*) is currently recommended as the best to detect a breast mass, but two other patterns are in common use: from the nipple palpating out to the periphery, as if following spokes on a wheel, and in concentric circles out to the periphery (see Fig. 10.5, *B* and *C*). In every pattern, take care to palpate every square centimetre of the breast and to examine the tail of Spence high into the axilla.

In nulliparous women, normal breast tissue feels firm, smooth, and elastic. After pregnancy, the tissue feels softer and looser. Premenstrual engorgement is normal due to increasing progesterone and consists of a slight enlargement, a tenderness to palpation, and a generalized nodularity; the lobes feel prominent and their margins are more distinct.

A firm transverse ridge of compressed tissue in the lower quadrants, the **inframammary ridge,** is especially noticeable in large breasts. Do not confuse it with an abnormal lump.

For the woman with large, pendulous breasts, you may palpate by using a bimanual technique (Fig. 10.6). The woman should sit up and lean forward. Support the inferior part of the breast with one hand. Use your other hand to palpate the breast tissue against your supporting hand.

Heat, redness, and swelling in nonlactating and nonpostpartum breasts indicate inflammation.

Normal Range of Findings	Abnormal Findings

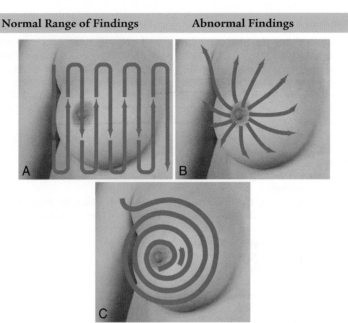

10.5   Patterns of breast palpation. **A.** Vertical strip pattern. **B.** Spokes-on-a-wheel pattern. **C.** Concentric circles pattern.

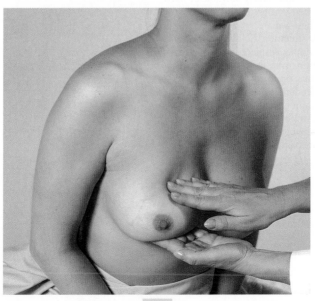

10.6

Continued

Normal Range of Findings	Abnormal Findings
Palpate the nipple. Note any induration or subareolar masses. Use your thumb and forefinger to gently depress the nipple tissue into the well behind the areola. The tissue should move inward easily. If any discharge appears, note its colour and consistency. Pressing a white gauze pad to the discharge helps to determine its colour.	Discharge is abnormal, except in pregnancy and lactation. (See Table 18.6, p. 444, in Jarvis: *Physical Examination and Health Assessment,* 3rd Canadian edition.) Test any abnormal discharge for the presence of blood.
If you feel a lump or mass, note these characteristics:	
1. Location: Using the breast as a clock face, describe the distance in centimetres from the nipple (e.g., "7:00 position, 2 cm from the nipple"). Or diagram the breast in the woman's record and mark the location of the lump.	See Table 10.1, for descriptions of common breast lumps with these characteristics.
2. Size: In centimetres, in three dimensions: width × length × thickness.	
3. Shape: Oval, round, lobulated, or indistinct.	
4. Consistency: Soft, firm, or hard.	
5. Movable: Freely movable or fixed when you try to slide it over the chest wall.	
6. Distinctness: Solitary or multiple.	
7. Nipple: Displaced or retracted.	
8. Skin over the lump: Erythematous, dimpled, or retracted.	
9. Tenderness: Note whether the lump is tender to palpation.	
10. Lymphadenopathy: Determine whether any regional lymph nodes are palpable.	

Normal Range of Findings	Abnormal Findings

Teach Breast Self-Examination

According to the Canadian Cancer Society (2017a) "There really isn't a right or wrong way for women to examine their breasts. They just need to know the whole area of their breast tissue well enough to notice changes. This includes the entire breast area up to the collarbone and under the armpits, as well as the nipples." Reinforce to patients that self-examination will familiarize them with their own breasts and their normal variation. Emphasize the absence of lumps (not the presence of them). However, do encourage women to report any unusual finding promptly.

Keep your teaching simple; the simpler the plan, the more likely the patient is to comply. Suggest that women inspect their breasts in front of a mirror while disrobed to the waist. Encourage women to learn how their breasts feel while in the shower, where soap and water assist palpation, and while lying supine so that breast tissue is flattened. Encourage each woman to palpate her own breasts while you are there to monitor her technique. Use the return demonstration to assess the patient's technique and understanding of the procedure.

The Breast Examination in Men

Inspect the chest wall, noting the skin surface and any lumps or swelling. Palpate the nipple area for any lumps or tissue enlargement. It should feel even, with no nodules. Palpate the axillary lymph nodes.

Of all new cases of cancer in men per year, breast cancer represented 0.2% in 2016 (Canadian Cancer Statistics Advisory Committee, 2017).

Continued

Normal Range of Findings	Abnormal Findings

The normal male breast has a flat disc of undeveloped breast tissue beneath the nipple. **Gynecomastia** is an enlargement of this breast tissue, making it clinically distinguishable from the other tissue in the chest wall. It feels like a smooth, firm, movable disc. This occurs normally during puberty. It usually affects only one breast and is temporary.

Gynecomastia also occurs with use of anabolic steroids, some medications, and in some disease states. (See Table 18.8, p. 446, in Jarvis: *Physical Examination and Health Assessment,* 3rd Canadian edition.)

 ## DEVELOPMENTAL CONSIDERATIONS

Infants and Children

In the neonate, the breasts may be enlarged and may secrete a clear or white fluid called "witch's milk." These signs are not significant and are resolved within a few days to a few weeks.

Adolescents

Adolescent breast development usually begins between 8 and 10 years of age. Expect some asymmetry during growth as a normal finding. (Distinguish breast development from extra adipose tissue present in obese children.) Full development takes an average of 3 years, with a range of 1.5 to 6 years.

Note precocious development occurring before age 8 years. It is usually normal, but also occurs with thyroid dysfunction, stilbestrol ingestion, or ovarian or adrenal tumour.

Note delayed development occurring with hormonal failure, anorexia nervosa beginning before puberty, or severe malnutrition.

With the maturing adolescent, palpate the breasts as you would with the adult. The breasts normally feel firm and uniform. Note any mass.

At this age, a mass is almost always a benign **fibroadenoma** or a cyst.

Normal Range of Findings	Abnormal Findings

Pregnant Women

A delicate, blue vascular pattern is visible over the breasts. The breasts increase in size, as do the nipples. Jagged linear stretch marks, or striae, may develop if the breasts have a marked increase in size. The nipples also become darker and more erectile. The areolae widen, grow darker, and contain small, scattered, elevated Montgomery's glands. On palpation, the breasts feel more nodular, and thick yellow colostrum can be expressed after the first trimester.

Lactating Women

Colostrum changes to milk production around the third postpartum day. At this time, the breasts may become engorged; appear enlarged, reddened, and shiny; and feel warm and hard. Frequent nursing helps drain the ducts and sinuses and stimulates milk production.

Nipple soreness is normal, occurs after the baby feeds for approximately the first 20 times, lasts 24 to 48 hours, then disappears rapidly. The nipples may look red and irritated, and may even crack, but they heal rapidly if kept dry and exposed to air. Frequent nursing is the best treatment for nipple soreness.

If one section of the breast surface appears red and tender, a duct is plugged. (See Table 18.7, p. 445, in Jarvis: *Physical Examination and Health Assessment,* 3rd Canadian edition.)

Older Women

The breasts look pendulous, flattened, and sagging. Nipples may be retracted, but can be pulled outward. The breasts feel more granular, and the terminal ducts around the nipple feel more prominent and stringy. Thickening of the inframammary ridge at the lower breast is normal and feels more prominent with age.

Reinforce the value of routine breast health behaviours. Women older than 50 years of age have an increased risk of breast cancer (see Table 10.2).

Because atrophy causes shrinkage of normal glandular tissue, cancer detection is somewhat easier. Any palpable lump not positively identified as a normal structure should be investigated.

Continued

Summary Checklist: Breasts and Regional Lymphatic Examination

1. **Inspect breasts** as the woman sits, raises arms over head, pushes hands on hips, and leans forward
2. **Inspect** the **supraclavicular and infraclavicular areas**
3. **Palpate** the **axillae** and **regional lymph nodes**
4. With woman supine, **palpate the breast tissue,** including the tail of Spence, the nipples, and the areolae
5. **Engage in teaching and health promotion**

ABNORMAL FINDINGS

TABLE 10.1	Breast Lump

Benign Breast Disease

Multiple tender masses. Formerly called *fibrocystic breast disease*; this is a meaningless term because it covers too many entities. Actually, six diagnostic categories exist, based on symptoms and physical findings (Love & Lindsey, 2015):

- Swelling and tenderness (cyclical discomfort)
- Mastalgia (severe pain, both cyclical and noncyclical)
- Nodularity (significant lumpiness, both cyclical and noncyclical)
- Dominant lumps (including cysts and fibroadenomas)
- Nipple discharge (including intraductal papilloma and duct ectasia)
- Infections and inflammations (including subareolar abscess, lactational mastitis, breast abscess, and Mondor's disease)

About 50% of all women have some form of benign breast disease. Nodularity occurs bilaterally; nodules are regular, firm, mobile, well demarcated, and feel rubbery, like small water balloons. Pain may be dull, heavy, and cyclical, or may occur just before menses as nodules enlarge. Some women have nodularity but no pain, or vice versa. Cysts are discrete, fluid-filled sacs. Dominant lumps and nipple discharge must be investigated carefully and may need to undergo biopsy to rule out cancer. Nodularity itself is not premalignant, but may cause difficulty in detecting truly cancerous lumps.

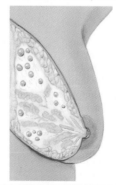

TABLE 10.1	Breast Lump—cont'd

Cancer

Solitary unilateral nontender mass. Single focus in one area, although it may be interspersed with other nodules. Solid, hard, dense, and fixed to underlying tissues or skin as cancer becomes invasive. Borders are irregular and poorly delineated. Grows constantly. Often painless, but may cause pain. Most common in upper outer quadrant. Usually found in women 30–80 years of age; risk increases at ages 50–69 years. As cancer advances, signs include firm or hard irregular axillary nodes, skin dimpling, and nipple retraction, elevation, and discharge.

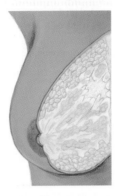

Fibroadenoma

Solitary nontender benign mass. Most common between 15 and 30 years of age, but can occur up to age 55 years; is most commonly self-detected in late adolescence. Solid, firm, rubbery, and elastic. Round, oval or lobulated; 1–5 cm. Freely movable, slippery; fingers slide it easily through tissue. Usually no axillary lymphadenopathy. Diagnosis is based on history, physical examination, ultrasonography; suspect tumours (i.e., large, rapidly growing, or other suspect findings) may necessitate biopsy, surgical excision, or both (Jayasinghe & Simmons, 2009).

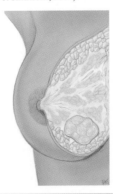

TABLE 10.2	Risk Factors for Breast Cancer	
Unmodifiable Risk Factors	Modifiable Risk Factors	Possible Risk Factors*
Female sex, age between 50 and 69 years	Nulliparity or first child after age 30 years	Physical inactivity
Personal history of breast cancer	Hormonal contraceptive use	Adult weight gain
Family history of breast cancer	Hormone replacement therapy	Smoking and second-hand smoke exposure
Dense breasts	Alcohol intake of ≥1 drink daily	High birth weight
BRCA gene mutation	Obesity	Night shift work
Ashkenazi Jewish ancestry	High socioeconomic status	Certain benign breast conditions
Specific rare genetic conditions		
Early menarche (before age 11 years) or late menopause (age 55 or older)		
Exposure to ionizing radiation		
Atypical hyperplasia		
Tall adult height		

*Although possible risk factors have some association with breast cancer, evidence at the time of publication is insufficient to identify these as known risk factors.
Data adapted from Canadian Cancer Society. (2018). *Risk factors for breast cancer*. Retrieved from http://www.cancer.ca/en/cancer-information/cancer-type/breast/risks/?region=on.

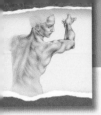

CHAPTER | 11

Thorax and Lungs

STRUCTURE AND FUNCTION

The **thoracic cage** is a bony structure with a conical shape (Fig. 11.1). It is defined by the sternum, 12 pairs of **ribs**, 12 thoracic **vertebrae**, and the **diaphragm**.

The *costochondral junctions* are the points at which the ribs join their cartilages. They are not palpable.

The *suprasternal notch* is the hollow U-shaped depression just above the sternum, in between the clavicles.

The *sternal angle,* or *angle of Louis,* is the articulation of the manubrium and body of the sternum, and it is continuous with the second rib. Each intercostal space is numbered by the rib above it.

The *costal angle* is formed by the right and left costal margins where they meet at the xiphoid process. It is usually 90 degrees or less.

The **trachea** lies anterior to the esophagus and is 10 to 11 cm long in adults (Fig. 11.2). It begins at the level of the cricoid cartilage in the neck and bifurcates just below the sternal angle into the right and left main bronchi.

An **acinus** is a functional respiratory unit and consists of the bronchioles and alveoli. Gaseous exchange occurs across the respiratory membrane in the alveolar duct and in the millions of alveoli.

In the anterior chest, the **apex,** or highest point, of lung tissue is 3 or 4 cm above the inner third of the clavicles (Fig. 11.3). The **base,** or

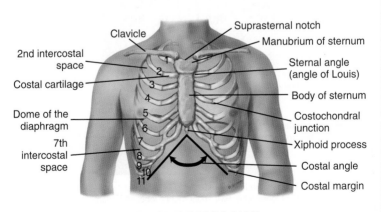

ANTERIOR THORACIC CAGE

11.1 Anterior thoracic cage. *(© Pat Thomas, 2010.)*

123

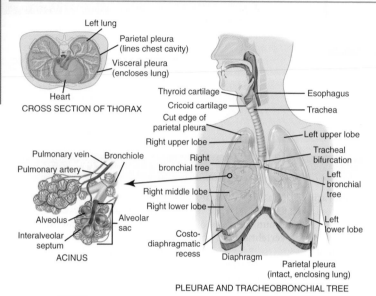

Left lung

Parietal pleura
(lines chest cavity)

Visceral pleura
(encloses lung)

Heart

CROSS SECTION OF THORAX

Thyroid cartilage

Cricoid cartilage

Cut edge of
parietal pleura

Right upper lobe

Esophagus

Trachea

Left upper lobe

Tracheal
bifurcation

Left
bronchial
tree

Left
lower lobe

Pulmonary vein — Bronchiole

Pulmonary artery

Right
bronchial tree

Right middle lobe

Right lower lobe

Alveolus

Interalveolar
septum

Alveolar
sac

ACINUS

Costo-
diaphragmatic
recess

Diaphragm

Parietal pleura
(intact, enclosing lung)

PLEURAE AND TRACHEOBRONCHIAL TREE

11.2   Pleurae and tracheobronchial tree. *(© Pat Thomas, 2010.)*

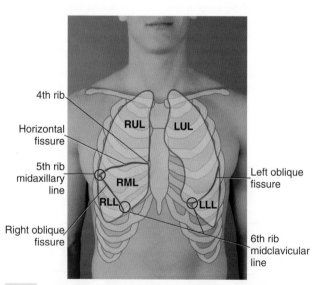

4th rib

Horizontal
fissure

5th rib
midaxillary
line

Right oblique
fissure

RUL   LUL

RML

RLL

LLL

Left oblique
fissure

6th rib
midclavicular
line

11.3   Lobes of the lungs—anterior. *LLL*, left lower lobe; *LUL*, left upper lobe; *RLL*, right lower lobe; *RML*, right middle lobe; *RUL*, right upper lobe.

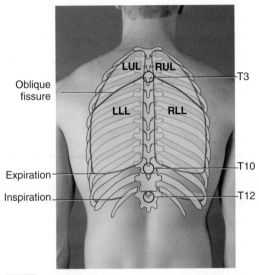

11.4 Lobes of the lungs—posterior. *LLL*, left lower lobe; *LUL*, left upper lobe; *RLL*, right lower lobe; *RUL*, right upper lobe.

lower border, rests on the diaphragm. The right lung has three lobes, and the left lung has two lobes. The lobes are separated by **fissures.**

Posteriorly, the location of the seventh cervical vertebra (C7) marks the apex of lung tissue and T10 usually corresponds to the base (Fig. 11.4). The most remarkable point about the posterior chest is that its contents consist almost entirely of lower lobe. The upper lobes occupy only a small band of tissue from the apices down to T3 or T4. The rest is all lower lobe. The right middle lobe does not project onto the posterior chest.

SOCIAL DETERMINANTS OF HEALTH CONSIDERATIONS

In 2015, 1639 new active and re-emergent cases of tuberculosis (TB) were reported to the Canadian Tuberculosis Reporting System. Since 2005, the total number of reported cases of active **tuberculosis** disease has remained relatively stable. The western provinces, territories, and Nunavut share the highest incidence in the country, with foreign-born individuals and Canadians of Indigenous descent disproportionately represented among reported cases of TB. Pulmonary TB remained the most commonly reported site of disease. Low socioeconomic conditions, number of household inhabitants, and access to health care resources all impact both the ability to diagnose and subsequently treat the condition; 84% of all Canadians diagnosed in 2015 were successfully treated (Gallant, Duccuri, & McGuire, 2017). In 2014, 2.4 million people reported that they had been diagnosed with **asthma** by a health professional. This rate has remained fairly consistent since 2001. The two most important preventable risk factors for respiratory disease are tobacco smoke (both personal and second-hand) and poor air quality (indoor and outdoor). Asthma was a contributing factor in approximately 10% of the hospital admissions of children younger than 5 years and in 8% of those aged 5 to 14 years (Tarlo & Lemiere, 2014).

Respiratory diseases, including lung cancer, are a major cause of death in Canada. Lung cancer remains the leading cause of cancer death in both men and women. In 2017, the Canadian Cancer Society estimated that one per 11 men is expected to develop lung cancer during his lifetime, and 1 per 14 will die of it. One per 14 women is expected to develop lung cancer during her lifetime, and 1 per 17 is expected to die of it. The incidence rate among women, although still elevated, appears to be stabilizing. In men, the incidence has been decreasing (Canadian Cancer Society, 2017).

SUBJECTIVE DATA

1. Cough (duration, productive of sputum)
2. Shortness of breath (with level of activity)
3. Chest pain with breathing
4. Past history of respiratory disease (bronchitis, emphysema, asthma, pneumonia, tuberculosis)
5. Smoking history (number of packs per day, number of years smoked)
6. Environmental exposure that affects breathing (e.g., occupational hazard, urban environment)
7. Self-care behaviours (last tuberculin skin test, chest x-ray, influenza immunization)

OBJECTIVE DATA

PREPARATION

Ask the patient to sit upright and to leave the gown on and open at the back.

EQUIPMENT NEEDED

Stethoscope
Small ruler marked in centimetres
Marking pen
Alcohol wipe (to clean end piece)

Normal Range of Findings	Abnormal Findings
Inspect the Posterior Chest	
Shape and Configuration. The spinous processes should appear in a straight line. The thorax is symmetrical, in an elliptical shape, with downward sloping ribs. The scapulae are placed symmetrically.	Skeletal deformities may limit thoracic cage excursions, including scoliosis (S-shaped curvature) and kyphosis (outward curvature) of the thoracic spine.
The anteroposterior diameter of the chest should be less than the transverse diameter. The normal ratio of anteroposterior to transverse diameter is approximately 1:2.	Anteroposterior diameter equals transverse diameter ("barrel chest"). Ribs are horizontal, chest appears as if held in continuous inspiration. This occurs in chronic emphysema as a result of hyperinflation of the lungs.

Normal Range of Findings	Abnormal Findings

The neck muscles and trapezius muscles should have developed normally for age and occupation.

Neck muscles are hypertrophied in chronic obstructive pulmonary disease (COPD) as a result of aiding in forced respirations.

Position. This includes a relaxed posture and the ability to support his or her own weight with arms comfortably at the sides or hands in the lap.

With COPD, a tripod position (leaning forward with arms braced against knees, chair, or bed) gives leverage so that the rectus abdominis, intercostal, and accessory neck muscles all can aid in expiration.

Skin Colour and Condition. Colour should be consistent with patient's genetic background, with no cyanosis or pallor. Note any lesions.

Cyanosis occurs with tissue hypoxia.

Palpate the Posterior Chest

Symmetrical Expansion. Confirm *symmetrical chest expansion* by placing your warmed hands on the posterolateral chest wall with thumbs at the level of T9 or T10. Slide your hands medially to pinch up a small fold of skin between your thumbs. Ask the patient to take a deep breath; your thumbs should move apart symmetrically. Note any lag in expansion.

Unequal chest expansion occurs with marked atelectasis or pneumonia, with thoracic trauma, such as fractured ribs, or with pneumothorax.

Pain accompanies deep breathing when the pleurae are inflamed.

Tactile Fremitus. *Tactile* (or *vocal*) *fremitus* is a palpable vibration. Use the palmar base (the ball) of the fingers or the ulnar edge of one hand and touch the patient's chest while he or she repeats the words "ninety-nine" or "blue moon." Start over the lung apices and palpate from one side to another; the vibrations should feel the same in the corresponding area on each side. Fremitus is most prominent between the scapulae and around the sternum, sites where the major bronchi are closest to the chest wall. It normally decreases as you progress down because more and more tissue impedes sound transmission.

Decreased fremitus occurs when anything obstructs transmission of vibrations (e.g., obstructed bronchus, pleural effusions or thickening, pneumothorax, or emphysema).

Increased fremitus occurs with compression or consolidation of lung tissue (e.g., lobar pneumonia).

Rhonchal fremitus is palpable with thick bronchial secretions.

Pleural friction fremitus is palpable with inflammation of the pleura. (See Table 19.6, p. 482, in Jarvis: *Physical Examination and Health Assessment,* 3rd Canadian edition.)

Chest Wall. Using the fingers, gently *palpate the entire chest wall.* Note any areas of tenderness, the skin temperature and moisture, any superficial lumps or masses, and any skin lesions.

Crepitus is a coarse, crackling sensation palpable over the skin surface. It occurs in subcutaneous emphysema when air escapes from the lung and enters the subcutaneous tissue, as after open thoracic injury or surgery.

Continued

Normal Range of Findings	Abnormal Findings

Percuss the Posterior Chest

Lung Fields. Start at the apices and percuss the band of normally resonant tissue across the tops of both shoulders. Then percuss in the interspaces, making a side-to-side comparison all the way down the lung region. Percuss at 5-cm intervals. Avoid the scapulae and ribs.

Resonance. Resonance is the low-pitched, clear, hollow sound that predominates in healthy lung tissue in the adult. The resonant note may be modified somewhat in athletes with heavily muscular chest walls and in obese adults, in whom subcutaneous fat produces scattered dullness.

Diaphragmatic Excursion. Percuss to map out the lower lung border, both in expiration and inspiration. Measure the difference. This *diaphragmatic excursion* should be equal bilaterally and measure about 3 to 5 cm in adults, although it may be up to 7 to 8 cm in well-conditioned people.

Hyperresonance is a lower-pitched, booming sound found when too much air is present, as in emphysema or pneumothorax.

A **dull note** (soft, muffled thud) signals abnormal density in the lungs, as with pneumonia, pleural effusion, atelectasis, or tumour.

An abnormally high level of dullness on the chest wall, as well as absence of excursion, occurs with pleural effusion (fluid in the space between the visceral and parietal pleura) and atelectasis of the lower lobes.

Auscultate the Posterior Chest

Breath Sounds. Instruct the patient to breathe through the mouth a little bit deeper than usual. While standing behind the patient, listen to the following lung areas: posterior from the apices at C7 to the bases (around T10), and laterally from the axilla down to the seventh or eighth rib. Use the sequence illustrated in Fig. 11.5. You should expect to hear three types of normal breath sounds: **bronchial** (sometimes called *tracheal* or *tubular*), **bronchovesicular,** and **vesicular** (see Table 11.1).

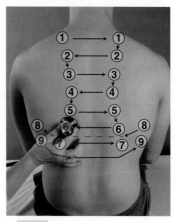

11.5 Sequence for auscultation.

Normal Range of Findings	Abnormal Findings

Normal Range of Findings

Note the normal location of the three types of breath sounds (Figs. 11.6 and 11.7).

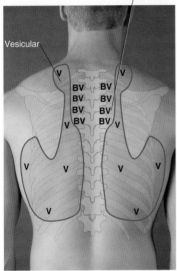

11.6 Breath sounds on the posterior chest.

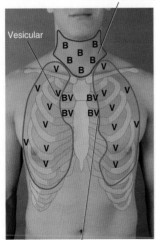

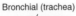

Bronchovesicular

11.7 Breath sounds on the anterior chest.

Abnormal Findings

Decreased or absent breath sounds occur:
1. When the bronchial tree is obstructed by secretions, mucous plug, or a foreign body.
2. In emphysema, as a result of loss of elasticity in the lung fibres and decreased force of inspired air.
3. When anything obstructs transmission of sound between the lung and your stethoscope, such as pleurisy or pleural thickening, or air (pneumothorax) or fluid (pleural effusion) in the pleural space.

Increased breath sounds are sounds louder than they should be (e.g., bronchial sounds are abnormal over the peripheral lung fields). They occur when consolidation (e.g., pneumonia) or compression (e.g., fluid in the intrapleural space) yields a denser lung area that enhances the transmission of sound from the bronchi. When the inspired air reaches the alveoli, it hits solid lung tissue, which conducts sound more efficiently to the surface.

Continued

Normal Range of Findings	Abnormal Findings

Adventitious Sounds. Note the presence of any *adventitious sounds.* These are abnormal sounds caused by the collision of moving air with secretions in the tracheobronchial passageways or by the popping open of previously deflated airways. If you hear adventitious sounds, be sure to describe whether they are on inspiration or expiration, their loudness, their pitch, and their location on the chest wall.

Crackles (or rales) are a result of pneumonia and pulmonary edema, and **wheezes** (or rhonchi) are a result of asthma and emphysema (see Table 11.2).

Inspect the Anterior Chest

Shape and Configuration. The ribs are sloping downward with symmetrical interspaces. The costal angle is within 90 degrees. Development of abdominal muscles is as expected for the patient's age, weight, and athletic condition.

Barrel chest is characterized by horizontal ribs and costal angle exceeding 90 degrees.

Hypertrophy of abdominal muscles occurs with chronic emphysema.

Facial Expression. Relaxed and benign, indicating unconscious effort of breathing.

Facies appear tense, strained, and tired in COPD.

Level of Consciousness. Alert and cooperative.

Cerebral hypoxia may be manifested by excessive drowsiness or by anxiety, restlessness, and irritability.

Skin Colour and Condition. The lips and nail beds are free of cyanosis or unusual pallor. The nails are of normal configuration.

Clubbing of the distal phalanx occurs with chronic respiratory disease.

Cutaneous angiomas (spider nevi) associated with liver disease or portal hypertension may be evident on the chest.

Quality of Respirations. Normal, relaxed breathing is automatic and effortless, regular, and even, and produces no noise. The chest expands symmetrically with each inspiration. Note any localized lag on inspiration.

Noisy breathing occurs with severe asthma or chronic bronchitis.

Unequal chest expansion occurs when part of the lung is obstructed or collapsed, as with pneumonia, or in guarding to avoid postoperative incisional pain or the pain of pleurisy.

Normally, accessory muscles are not used to augment respiratory effort.

The rectus abdominis and internal intercostal muscles are used to force expiration in COPD.

The respiratory rate is within normal limits for the patient's age, and the pattern of breathing is regular. Occasional sighs normally punctuate breathing.

Tachypnea and hyperventilation, bradypnea and hypoventilation, and periodic breathing are abnormal (see full description in Table 11.3).

Normal Range of Findings	Abnormal Findings

Percuss the Anterior Chest

Begin at the apices in the supraclavicular areas. Percussing the interspaces and comparing one side to the other, move down the anterior chest.

Note the borders of cardiac dullness normally found on the anterior chest, and do not confuse these with suspected lung pathology. In the right hemithorax, the upper border of liver dullness is located in the fifth intercostal space in the right midclavicular line. On the left, tympany is evident over the gastric space. (See Fig. 19.23, p. 473, in Jarvis: *Physical Examination and Health Assessment*, 3rd Canadian edition.)

Lungs are hyperinflated with chronic emphysema, resulting in hyperresonance, where cardiac dullness would be expected.

Auscultate the Anterior Chest

Auscultate the lung fields over the anterior chest from the apices in the supraclavicular areas down to the sixth rib. Progress from side to side as you move downward, and listen to one full respiration in each location.

You should expect to hear vesicular breath sounds over most of the anterior lung fields as indicated in Fig. 11.7.

 DEVELOPMENTAL CONSIDERATIONS

Infants and Children

Count the respiratory rate for 1 full minute when the infant is asleep, if possible, because infants reach rapid rates with very little excitation when awake. The respiratory pattern may be irregular when there are extremes in room temperature or with feeding or sleeping. Brief periods of apnea less than 10 or 15 seconds are common. This periodic breathing is more common in premature infants.

Auscultation normally yields bronchovesicular breath sounds in the peripheral lung fields in the infant and young child up to age 5 or 6 years, because of the relatively thin chest wall with underdeveloped musculature.

Rapid respiratory rates accompany pneumonia, fever, pain, heart disease, and anemia.

In an infant, tachypnea (rate of 50 to 100 breaths per minute during sleep) may be an early sign of heart failure.

Diminished breath sounds occur with pneumonia, atelectasis, pleural effusion, or pneumothorax.

Continued

Normal Range of Findings	Abnormal Findings
Fine crackles are the adventitious sounds commonly heard in the immediate neonatal period as a result of the opening of the airways and clearing of fluid. Because the newborn's chest wall is so thin, transmission of sounds is enhanced and heard easily all over the chest, making localizations of breath sounds difficult. Even bowel sounds are easily heard in the chest. Try using the smaller pediatric diaphragm end piece of a stethoscope, or place the bell over the infant's interspaces and not over the ribs.	Persistent fine crackles scattered over the chest occur with pneumonia, bronchiolitis, or atelectasis. Crackles only in upper lung fields occur with cystic fibrosis; crackles only in lower lung fields occur with heart failure. Expiratory wheezing occurs with lower airway obstruction (e.g., asthma or bronchiolitis). Persistent peristaltic sounds with diminished breath sounds on the same side may indicate diaphragmatic hernia. Stridor is a high-pitched inspiratory crowing sound heard without the stethoscope that occurs with upper airway obstruction (e.g., croup, foreign body aspiration, or acute epiglottitis).

Pregnant Women

The thoracic cage may appear wider, and the costal angle widens by about 50%. Respirations may be deeper, with a 40% increase in tidal volume.

Older Adults

The thoracic cage commonly has an increased anteroposterior diameter, giving a round barrel shape, and **kyphosis,** an outward curvature of the thoracic spine. The patient compensates by holding the head extended and tilted back.

You may palpate marked bony prominences because of decreased subcutaneous fat. Chest expansion may be somewhat decreased although still symmetrical. The costal cartilages become calcified with age, resulting in a less mobile thorax.

An older patient may fatigue easily, especially during auscultation when deep mouth breathing is required. Take care that this patient does not hyperventilate and become dizzy. Allow brief rest periods or quiet breathing. If the patient does feel faint, holding the breath for a few seconds will restore equilibrium.

Summary Checklist: Thorax and Lung Examination

1. **Inspection:**
   Assess thoracic cage
   Measure respirations
   Assess skin colour and
     condition
   Evaluate patient's position
   Observe patient's facial
     expression
   Assess level of consciousness
2. **Palpation:**
   Confirm symmetrical expansion
   Assess tactile fremitus
   Detect any lumps, masses,
     tenderness

3. **Percussion:**
   Percuss over lung fields
   Estimate diaphragmatic excursion
4. **Auscultation:**
   Assess normal breath sounds
   Note any abnormal breath
     sounds
   If breath sounds are abnormal,
     perform bronchophony,
     whispered pectoriloquy, and
     egophony
   Note any adventitious sounds
5. **Engage in teaching and health
   promotion**

ABNORMAL FINDINGS

TABLE 11.1	Characteristics of Normal Breath Sounds				
Type of Breath Sound	Pitch	Amplitude	Duration	Quality	Normal Location
Bronchial (Tracheal)	High	Loud	Inspiration < expiration	Harsh, hollow, tubular	Trachea and larynx
Bronchovesicular	Moderate	Moderate	Inspiration = expiration	Mixed	Over major bronchi, where fewer alveoli are located: posterior, be-tween scapulae especially on right; anterior, around upper sternum in first and second in-tercostal space
Vesicular	Low	Soft	Inspiration > expiration	Rustling, like the sound of the wind in the trees	Over peripheral lung fields, where air flows through smaller bron-chioles and alveoli

TABLE 11.2	Adventitious Lung Sounds		
Sound	Description	Mechanism	Clinical Example
Discontinuous Sounds			
These are discrete, crackling sounds.			
Crackles: fine (formerly called rales) Inspiration Expiration	Discontinuous, high-pitched, short, crackling, popping sounds heard during inspiration that are not cleared by coughing.	Inhaled air collides with previously deflated airways; airways suddenly pop open, creating crackling sound as gas pressures between the two compartments equalize.	*Late inspiratory crackles* occur with restrictive disease: pneumonia, congestive heart failure, and interstitial fibrosis. *Early inspiratory crackles* occur with obstructive disease: chronic bronchitis, asthma, and emphysema. *Posturally induced crackles (PICs)* are fine crackles that appear with a change from sitting to the supine position or with a change from supine to supine with legs elevated. PICs that appear after acute myocardial infarction have been associated with increased mortality.
Crackles: coarse 	Loud, low-pitched, bubbling, and gurgling sounds that start in early inspiration and may be present in expiration; may decrease somewhat after suctioning or coughing but will reappear shortly.	Inhaled air collides with secretions in the trachea and large bronchi.	Pulmonary edema, pneumonia, pulmonary fibrosis, and a depressed cough reflex in terminally ill patients.
Atelectatic crackles (atelectatic rales) 	Sound like fine crackles but do not last and are not indications of disease. Disappear after the first few breaths. Heard in axillae and bases (usually dependent) of lungs.	When sections of alveoli are not fully aerated, they deflate and accumulate secretions. Crackles are heard when these sections re-expand with a few deep breaths.	Occur in older adults, bedridden patients, or in patients just aroused from sleep.

TABLE 11.2 Adventitious Lung Sounds—cont'd

Sound	Description	Cause
Pleural friction rub	A very superficial sound that is coarse and low pitched; it has a grating quality as if two pieces of leather are being rubbed together. Sounds just like crackles, but *close* to the ear. Sound is inspiratory and expiratory.	Caused when pleurae become inflamed and lose their normal lubricating fluid. Their opposing, roughened pleural surfaces rub together during respiration.	Pleuritis, accompanied by pain with breathing. (Rub disappears after a few days if pleural fluid accumulates and separates pleurae.)

Continuous Sounds
These are connected, musical sounds.

Sound	Description	Cause
Wheeze: high-pitched (sibilant)	High-pitched, musical squeaking sounds that sound polyphonic (multiple notes as in a musical chord); predominate in expiration but may occur in both expiration and inspiration.	Air squeezed or compressed through passageways narrowed almost to closure by collapsing, swelling, secretions, or tumours.	Diffuse airway obstruction from acute asthma or chronic emphysema.
Wheeze: low-pitched (sonorous rhonchi)	Low-pitched, monophonic single note, musical snoring, moaning sounds. They are heard throughout the cycle, although they are more prominent on expiration. May clear somewhat after coughing.	Airflow obstruction. The pitch of the wheeze cannot be correlated to the size of the passageway that generates it.	Bronchitis, single bronchus obstruction from airway tumour.
Stridor	High-pitched, monophonic, inspiratory crowing sound, louder in neck than over chest wall.	Originating in larynx or trachea; upper airway obstruction from swollen, inflamed tissues or lodged foreign body.	Croup, and acute epiglottitis in children, foreign body inhalation, and obstructed airway (all may be life-threatening).

TABLE 11.3	Respiration Patterns*

Normal Adult (for Comparison)

Rate: 10–20 breaths per minute.

Depth—500–800 mL; air moving in and out with each respiration.

Pattern—even.

The ratio of pulse to respiration is fairly constant, about 4:1. Both values increase as a normal response to exercise, fear, or fever.

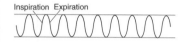

Tachypnea

Rapid shallow breathing. Increased rate is >24 per minute. This is a normal response to fever, fear, or exercise. Rate also increases with respiratory insufficiency, pneumonia, alkalosis, pleurisy, and lesions in the pons.

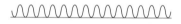

Bradypnea

Slow breathing. A decreased but regular rate (<10 per minute), as in drug-induced depression of the respiratory centre in the medulla, increased intracranial pressure, and diabetic coma.

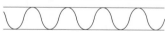

Sigh

Occasional sighs punctuate the normal breathing pattern and expand alveoli. Frequent sighs may indicate emotional dysfunction and may lead to hyperventilation and dizziness.

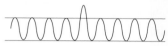

Hyperventilation

Increase in both rate and depth. Normally occurs with extreme exertion, fear, or anxiety. Also occurs with diabetic ketoacidosis (Kussmaul's respirations), hepatic coma, salicylate overdose (hyperventilation produces a respiratory alkalosis to compensate for the metabolic acidosis), lesions of the midbrain, and alteration in blood gas concentration (either an increase in carbon dioxide or decrease in oxygen). Hyperventilation causes the level of carbon dioxide in the blood to decrease (alkalosis).

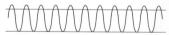

Hypoventilation

An irregular, shallow pattern caused by an overdose of narcotics or anaesthetics. May also occur with prolonged bed rest or conscious splinting of the chest to avoid respiratory pain.

TABLE 11.3	Respiration Patterns—cont'd

Cheyne-Stokes Respiration

A cycle in which respirations gradually increase in rate and depth and then decrease. The breathing periods last 30–45 seconds with periods of apnea (20 seconds) alternating the cycle. The most common cause is severe congestive heart failure; other causes are renal failure, meningitis, drug overdose, increased intracranial pressure. Occurs normally in infants and older adults during sleep.

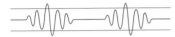

Chronic Obstructive Breathing

Normal inspiration and prolonged expiration to overcome increased airway resistance. In a patient with chronic obstructive lung disease, any situation calling for increased heart rate (exercise) may lead to dyspneic episode (air trapping) because then the patient does not have enough time for full expiration.

Normal   Prolonged
inspiration expiration   Air trapping

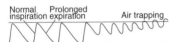

Biot's Respiration

Similar to Cheyne-Stokes respiration except that pattern is irregular. A series of normal respirations (three or four) is followed by a period of apnea. The cycle length is variable, lasting anywhere from 10 seconds to 1 minute. Occurs with head trauma, brain abscess, heatstroke, spinal meningitis, and encephalitis.

*Assess the (a) rate, (b) depth (tidal volume), and (c) pattern.

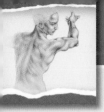

CHAPTER 12

Heart and Neck Vessels

STRUCTURE AND FUNCTION

The **precordium** is the area on the anterior chest overlying the heart and great vessels. The heart extends from the levels of the second to the fifth intercostal spaces and from the right border of the sternum to the left midclavicular line (Fig. 12.1).

Think of the heart as an upside-down triangle in the chest. The "top" of the heart is the broader *base,* and the "bottom" is the *apex,* which points down and to the left. During contraction, the apex beats against the chest wall, producing an apical impulse.

The right side of the heart pumps blood into the lungs, and the left side of the heart simultaneously pumps blood into the body. Each side has an **atrium** and a **ventricle** (Fig. 12.2).

The atrium is a thin-walled reservoir for holding blood, and the thick-walled ventricle is the muscular pumping chamber.

There are four **valves** in the heart. The two **atrioventricular (AV) valves** separate the atria and the ventricles. The right AV valve is the **tricuspid valve;** the left AV valve is the **bicuspid** or **mitral valve.** The AV valves open during the heart's filling phase, or diastole, to allow the ventricles to fill with blood.

The **semilunar valves** are located between the ventricles and the arteries. The semilunar valves are the **pulmonic valve** in the right side of the heart and the **aortic valve** in the left side of the heart. They open during

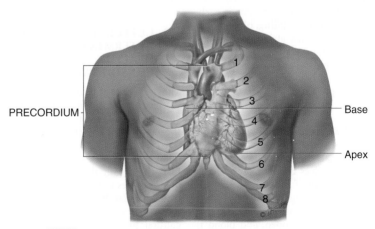

PRECORDIUM

Base

Apex

1
2
3
4
5
6
7
8

12.1 Position of the heart and great vessels. (© Pat Thomas, 2006.)

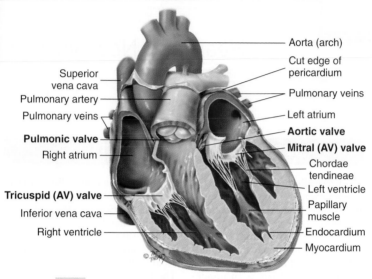

12.2 Heart wall, chambers, and valves. (© *Pat Thomas, 2006.*)

pumping, or **systole,** to allow blood to be ejected from the heart.

The **cardiac cycle** is the rhythmic movement of blood through the heart. It has two phases, diastole, and systole (Fig. 12.3).

In **diastole,** the ventricles relax and fill with blood. The AV valves, the tricuspid and mitral, are open. During the first rapid filling phase, **early or protodiastolic filling,** blood pours rapidly from the atria into the ventricles. Toward the end of diastole, the atria contract and push the last amount of blood into the ventricles, called **presystole** or **atrial systole** (sometimes referred to as the *atrial kick*).

The closure of the AV valves contributes to the first heart sound (S_1) and signals the beginning of **systole.** The AV valves close to prevent any regurgitation of blood back up into the atria during contraction. Then the semilunar valves, the aortic and pulmonic valves open, and blood is ejected rapidly into the arteries.

After the ventricles' contents are ejected, the semilunar valves close. This causes the second heart sound (S_2) and signals the end of systole.

Cardiovascular assessment includes the neck vessels: the carotid artery and the jugular veins (Fig. 12.4). These vessels reflect the efficiency of cardiac function.

CULTURAL AND SOCIAL DETERMINANTS OF HEALTH CONSIDERATIONS

The prevalence of death from cardiovascular disease (CVD) is sharply decreasing on an annual basis, and yet the incidence of CVD itself continues to increase. Canadians with the lowest household incomes were more likely than those with the highest household incomes to **report** living with a cardiovascular disease (Public Health Agency of Canada, 2016). Income, cultural food choices, and employment security are some of the

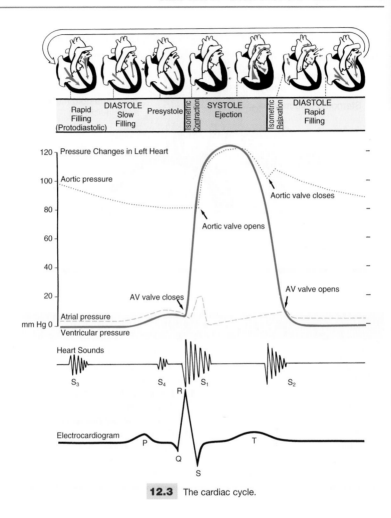

12.3   The cardiac cycle.

influencing factors that inhibit one's ability to manage CVD. Better medications, early intervention, and public health awareness are some of the factors contributing to the reduction in deaths.

Men and women in Canada have almost equal rates of death from CVD, a trend noted since 2000 (Government of Canada, 2017). Interestingly, as CVD death rates have diminished, rates of death from cancer have increased (29%), making cancer the number one killer of Canadians; it continues to rise annually (Government of Canada, 2018).

The prevalence of heart disease and stroke is higher among adults of African descent than in any other ethnic group (Statistics Canada, 2018). These differences in prevalence show the crucial need to improve early detection, screening, and treatment.

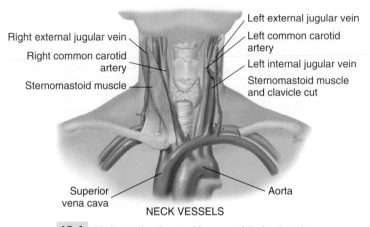

12.4   Neck vessels—the carotid artery and the jugular veins.

SUBJECTIVE DATA

1. Chest pain
2. Dyspnea
3. Orthopnea
4. Cough
5. Fatigue
6. Cyanosis or pallor
7. Edema
8. Nocturia
9. Past cardiac history (hypertension, elevated cholesterol or triglyceride levels, heart murmur, rheumatic fever, anemia, congenital heart disease)
10. Family cardiac history (hypertension, obesity, diabetes, coronary artery disease [CAD])
11. Personal habits (diet high in cholesterol, calories, or salt; smoking; alcohol use; drugs; amount of exercise; stress)

OBJECTIVE DATA

PREPARATION

To evaluate the carotid arteries, the patient can be sitting up. To assess the jugular veins and the precordium, the patient should be supine with the head and chest elevated between 30 and 40 degrees. Stand on the patient's right side.

EQUIPMENT NEEDED

Marking pen
Small ruler marked in centimetres
Stethoscope with diaphragm and bell end pieces
Alcohol wipe (to clean end pieces)

Normal Range of Findings	Abnormal Findings

The Neck Vessels

Auscultate the Carotid Artery

For patients older than middle age or who show symptoms or signs of CVD, auscultate each carotid artery for the presence of a **bruit.** This is a blowing, swishing sound indicating blood flow turbulence; normally, none is present.

A bruit indicates turbulence with a local vascular cause (e.g., atherosclerotic narrowing).

Keep the neck in a neutral position. Lightly apply the bell of the stethoscope over the carotid artery at three levels: (a) the angle of the jaw, (b) the midcervical area, and (c) the base of the neck. Avoid compressing the artery because this could create an artificial bruit. Ask the patient to hold his or her breath while you listen.

A carotid bruit is audible when the lumen is half to two-thirds occluded. Bruit loudness increases as the atherosclerosis worsens until the lumen is two-thirds occluded. When the lumen is completely occluded, the bruit disappears. Thus, absence of a bruit is not a sure indication of absence of a carotid lesion.

A murmur sounds much the same but is caused by a cardiac disorder. Some aortic valve murmurs (aortic stenosis) radiate to the neck and must be distinguished from a local bruit.

Palpate the Carotid Artery

Gently palpate **only one carotid artery at a time** to avoid compromising arterial blood to the brain.

Feel the contour and amplitude of the pulse. Normally the contour is smooth, with a rapid upstroke and slower downstroke, and the normal strength is moderate and equal bilaterally.

Diminished pulse feels small and weak (decreased stroke volume).

Increased pulse feels full and strong (hyperkinetic states; see Table 13.1, p. 165).

Inspect the Jugular Venous Pulse

Position the patient supine with the torso elevated anywhere from a 30- to a 45-degree angle. Remove the pillow to avoid flexing the neck. Turn the head slightly away from the examined side, and direct a strong light tangentially onto the neck to highlight pulsations and shadows.

NOTE: This inspection is considered by many authorities to be an advanced skill for practitioners in the cardiopulmonary environment, in particular. It is not considered part of the basic cardiac assessment when no other abnormal cardiac findings are evident.

Continued

Normal Range of Findings	Abnormal Findings
Note the external jugular veins overlying the sternomastoid muscle. In some patients, the veins are not visible at all; in others, they are full in the supine position. As the patient is raised to a sitting position, these external jugulars flatten and disappear, usually at 45 degrees.	Unilateral distension of external jugular veins has a local cause (e.g., kinking or aneurysm). Fully distended external jugular veins above 45 degrees signify increased central venous pressure (CVP), as with heart failure.

The Precordium

Inspect the Anterior Chest

You may or may not see the **apical impulse.** When visible, it appears at the level of the fourth or fifth intercostal space, at or inside the midclavicular line. It is easier to see in children and in patients with thin chest walls.

A **heave** or **lift** is a sustained forceful thrusting of the ventricle during systole. It occurs with ventricular hypertrophy and is seen at the sternal border (right ventricular heave) or the apex (left ventricular heave).

Palpate the Apical Impulse

Locate the apical impulse precisely by using one finger pad.

Note the following characteristics:
- Location: The apical impulse should occupy only one interspace, the fourth or fifth, and be at or medial to the midclavicular line
- Size: Normally 1 cm × 2 cm
- Amplitude: Normally a short, gentle tap
- Duration: Short, normally occupies only the first half of systole

The apical impulse is palpable in the supine position in 25% to 40% of adults and in the left lateral position in 50% to 73% of adults. It is not palpable in obese patients or patients with thick chest walls. With high cardiac output states (anxiety, fever, hyperthyroidism, anemia), the apical impulse increases in amplitude and duration.

Cardiac enlargement is characterized as follows:
- Left ventricular dilation (volume overload) displaces apical impulse down and to the left and increases size more than one space.
- Increased force and duration, but no change in location occurs with left ventricular hypertrophy, and no dilation (pressure overload).

Left ventricular dilation (volume overload) displaces the apical impulse down and to the left and increases size more than one costal vertebral space. This occurs with heart failure and cardiomyopathy.

Left ventricular hypertrophy presents with a sustained impulse, with increased force and duration, but no change in location.

Palpate Across the Precordium

Using the palmar aspects of your four fingers, gently palpate the apex, the left sternal border, and the base, searching for any other pulsations: normally none are felt. If any are present, note the timing. Use the carotid artery pulsation as a guide or auscultate as you palpate.

A **thrill** is a palpable vibration. It feels like the throat of a purring cat. The thrill signifies turbulent blood flow and accompanies loud murmurs. Absence of a thrill, however, does not necessarily rule out the presence of a murmur (see Table 12.2).

Normal Range of Findings	Abnormal Findings

Auscultation

Identify the auscultatory areas where you will listen. The four traditional valve "areas" (Fig. 12.5) are not over the actual anatomical locations of the valves, but are the sites on the chest wall where sounds produced by the valves are best heard:

- Second right interspace: aortic valve area
- Second left interspace: pulmonic valve area
- Fifth intercostal space at left lower sternal border: tricuspid valve area
- Fifth interspace at around left mid-clavicular line: mitral valve area

Do not limit your auscultation to only four locations because sounds produced by the valves may be heard all over the precordium. Learn to inch your stethoscope in a rough Z pattern, from the base of the heart across and down, then over to the apex; or, start at the apex and work your way up. Include the sites shown in Fig. 12.5.

Begin with the diaphragm end piece and use the following routine: (a) note the rate and rhythm; (b) identify S_1 and S_2; (c) assess S_1 and S_2 separately; (d) listen for extra heart sounds; and (e) listen for murmurs.

Note the Rate and Rhythm. The rate changes normally from 60 to 100 beats per minute. The rhythm should be regular, although **sinus arrhythmia** occurs normally in young adults and children. With sinus arrhythmia, the rhythm varies with the patient's breathing, increasing at the peak of inspiration and slowing with expiration. Note any other irregular rhythm.

Premature beat: An isolated beat is early or a pattern occurs in which every third or fourth beat sounds early.

Irregularly irregular: No pattern to the sounds; beats come rapidly and at random intervals.

Continued

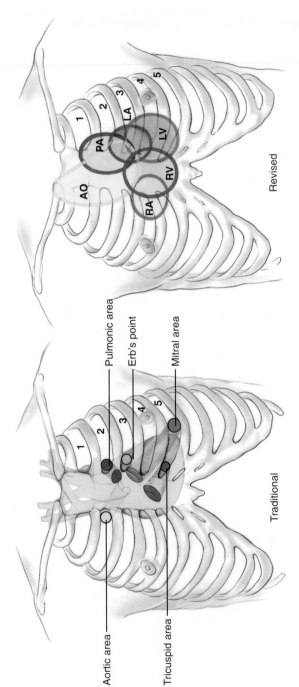

AUSCULTATORY AREAS

12.5 Auscultatory areas. *AO,* aorta; *LA,* left atrium; *LV,* left ventricle; *PA,* pulmonary artery; *RA,* right atrium; *RV,* right ventricle.

Normal Range of Findings	Abnormal Findings

Identify S₁ and S₂. Usually you can identify S_1 instantly because you hear a pair of sounds close together ("lub-dup"), and S_1 is the first of the pair. Other guidelines to distinguish S_1 from S_2 are as follows:

- S_1 is louder than S_2 at the apex; S_2 is louder than S_1 at the base.
- S_1 coincides with the carotid artery pulsation (Fig. 12.6).
- S_1 coincides with the R wave (the upstroke of the QRS complex) if the patient is on an ECG monitor.

Listen to S₁ and S₂ Separately. Note whether each heart sound is normal, accentuated, diminished, or split. Inch your diaphragm across the chest as you do this.

First Heart Sound (S₁). Caused by closure of the AV valves, S_1 signals the beginning of systole. You can hear it over the entire precordium, though it is loudest at the apex (Fig. 12.7).

Causes of accentuated or diminished **S₁**. (See Table 20.3, p. 526, in Jarvis: *Physical Examination and Health Assessment,* 3rd Canadian edition.)

Both heart sounds are diminished with increased air or tissue between the heart and your stethoscope, such as emphysema (hyperinflated lungs), obesity, and pericardial fluid.

Second Heart Sound (S₂). S_2 is associated with closure of the semilunar valves. You can hear it with the diaphragm over the entire precordium, although S_2 is loudest at the base (Fig. 12.8).

Accentuated or diminished **S₂**. (See Table 20.4, p. 527, in Jarvis: *Physical Examination and Health Assessment,* 3rd Canadian edition.)

Continued

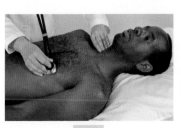

12.6

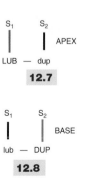

S₁   S₂
| | APEX
LUB — dup
12.7

S₁   S₂
| | BASE
lub — DUP
12.8

Normal Range of Findings	Abnormal Findings

Splitting of S₂. A split S_2 is a normal phenomenon that occurs toward the end of inspiration in some people. Recall that closure of the aortic and pulmonic valves is nearly synchronous. Because of the effects of respiration on the heart, inspiration separates the timing of the two valves' closure, and the aortic valve closes 0.06 second before the pulmonic valve. Instead of one "DUP," you hear a split sound: "T-DUP" (Fig. 12.9). During expiration, synchrony returns and the aortic and pulmonic components fuse together. A split S_2 is heard only in the pulmonic valve area (the second left interspace).

Concentrate on the split as you watch the patient's chest rise up and down with breathing. The split S_2 occurs about every fourth heartbeat, fading in with inhalation, and fading out with exhalation.

Focus on Systole, Then on Diastole, and Listen for Any Extra Heart Sounds. Listen with the diaphragm, then switch to the bell, covering all auscultatory areas. Usually these are silent periods. When you do detect an extra heart sound, listen carefully to note its timing and characteristics.

Listen for Murmurs. A murmur is a blowing, swooshing sound that occurs with turbulent blood flow in the heart or great vessels. Except for the innocent murmurs described, murmurs are abnormal. If you hear a murmur, describe it by indicating the following characteristics.

A **fixed split** is unaffected by respiration; the split is always there.

A **paradoxical split** is the opposite of what you would expect; the sounds fuse on inspiration and split on expiration. (See Table 20.5, p. 528, in Jarvis: *Physical Examination and Health Assessment,* 3rd Canadian edition.)

During systole, the **midsystolic click** (which is associated with mitral valve prolapse) is the most common extra sound. The S_3 and S_4 sounds occur in diastole; either may be normal or abnormal (Table 12.1).

Murmurs may be caused by congenital defects and acquired valvular defects. (See Tables 20.9 and 20.10, pages 533 and 534, in Jarvis: *Physical Examination and Health Assessment*, 3rd Canadian edition.)

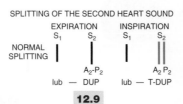

SPLITTING OF THE SECOND HEART SOUND

12.9

Normal Range of Findings	Abnormal Findings
Timing. Systole or diastole. Try to further describe the murmur as being in early, middle, or late systole or diastole; throughout the cardiac event (termed *pansystolic, holosystolic/ pandiastolic,* or *holodiastolic*); and whether it obscures or muffles the heart sounds.	A systolic murmur may occur with a normal heart or with heart disease; a diastolic murmur always indicates heart disease.
Loudness. The intensity in terms of six grades:	
Grade 1: Barely audible, heard only in a quiet room and then with difficulty	
Grade 2: Clearly audible, but faint	
Grade 3: Moderately loud, easy to hear	
Grade 4: Loud, associated with a thrill palpable on the chest wall	
Grade 5: Very loud, heard with one edge of the stethoscope lifted off the chest wall; associated thrill	
Grade 6: Loudest, still heard with entire stethoscope lifted just off the chest wall; associated thrill	
Pitch. High, medium, or low.	
Pattern. Growing louder (crescendo), tapering off (decrescendo), or increasing to a peak and then decreasing (crescendo–decrescendo, or diamond-shaped). Because the entire murmur is just milliseconds long, it takes practice to diagnose pattern.	
Quality. Musical, blowing, harsh, or rumbling.	The murmur of mitral stenosis is rumbling, whereas that of aortic stenosis is harsh.
Location. Area of maximum intensity of the murmur (where it is best heard) as noted by the valve area or intercostal spaces.	
Radiation. Heard in another place on the precordium, the neck, the back, or the axilla.	

Continued

Normal Range of Findings	Abnormal Findings

Posture. Murmurs may disappear or be enhanced by a change in position.

Some murmurs are common in healthy children or adolescents and are termed **innocent** or **functional**. The contractile force of the heart is greater in children. This increases blood flow velocity. The increased velocity, plus a smaller chest measurement, makes an audible murmur.

The innocent murmur is generally soft (grade 2), midsystolic, short, crescendo–decrescendo, and with a vibratory or musical quality ("vooot" sound). It is heard between the second or third left intercostal space and disappears with sitting, and the young patient has no associated signs of cardiac dysfunction.

Change Position. After auscultating in the supine position, roll the patient toward his or her left side. Listen with the bell at the apex for the presence of any diastolic filling sounds.

 DEVELOPMENTAL CONSIDERATIONS

Infants

Auscultate using the small (pediatric size) diaphragm and bell. The heart rate may range from 100 to 180 beats per minute immediately after birth, then stabilize to an average of 120 to 140 beats per minute. Infants normally have wide fluctuations with activity, from 170 beats per minute or more during crying or other activity to 70 to 90 beats per minute with sleeping.

Expect the heart rhythm to have sinus arrhythmia, the phasic speeding up or slowing down with the respiratory cycle.

Abnormal Findings column:

It is important to distinguish innocent murmurs from pathological ones. Diagnostic tests, such as electrocardiography (ECG) and echocardiography are needed to establish an accurate diagnosis.

S_3 and S_4 and the murmur of mitral stenosis are sometimes heard only when on the left side.

Persistent tachycardia:
- >200 per minute in newborns or
- >150 per minute in infants
Bradycardia:
- <90 per minute in newborns or
- <60 per minute in older infants or children
All warrant further investigation.

Investigate any irregularity, except sinus arrhythmia.

Normal Range of Findings	Abnormal Findings
Rapid rates make it more challenging to evaluate heart sounds. Expect heart sounds to be louder in infants than in adults because of the infant's thinner chest wall. S_2 has a higher pitch and is sharper than S_1. Splitting of S_2 just after the height of inspiration is common, not at birth, but beginning a few hours after birth.	Fixed split S_2 indicates atrial septal defect (ASD).
Murmurs in the immediate neonatal period do not necessarily indicate congenital heart disease. Murmurs are relatively common in the first 2 to 3 days because of fetal shunt closure. These murmurs are usually grades 1 or 2, systolic, accompany no other signs of cardiac disease, and disappear in 2 to 3 days. The murmur of patent ductus arteriosus (PDA) is a continuous machinery-like murmur, which disappears by 2 to 3 days.	
On the other hand, absence of a murmur in the immediate neonatal period does not ensure a perfect heart; congenital defects can be present that are not signalled by an early murmur. It is best to listen frequently and to note and describe any murmur according to the characteristics listed on p. 149.	Persistent murmur after 2 to 3 days, holosystolic murmurs, diastolic murmurs, and those that are loud all warrant further evaluation.
	For more information on murmurs due to congenital heart defects, see Table 20.9, p. 533, in Jarvis: *Physical Examination and Health Assessment*, 3rd Canadian edition.
Children Note any extracardiac or cardiac signs that may indicate heart disease.	Signs that indicate heart disease include poor weight gain, developmental delay, persistent tachycardia, tachypnea, dyspnea on exertion (DOE), cyanosis, and clubbing. Clubbing of fingers and toes does not appear until late in the first year, even with severe cyanotic defects.
The apical impulse is sometimes visible in children with thin chest walls.	Note any obvious bulge or any heave; these are **not** normal. A precordial bulge to the left of the sternum with a hyperdynamic precordium signals cardiac enlargement. The bulge occurs because the cartilaginous rib cage is more compliant. A substernal heave occurs with right ventricular enlargement, and an apical heave occurs with left ventricular hypertrophy.

Continued

Normal Range of Findings	Abnormal Findings
Palpate the apical impulse in the fourth intercostal space to the left of the midclavicular line until age 4 years; at the fourth interspace at the midclavicular line from ages 4 to 6 years; and in the fifth interspace to the right of the midclavicular line at age 7 years.	The apical impulse moves laterally with cardiac enlargement. Thrill (a palpable vibration).

The average heart rate slows as the child grows older, although it is still variable with rest or activity.

The heart rhythm remains characterized by sinus arrhythmia. Physiological S_3 is common in children (see Table 12.1). It occurs in early diastole, just after S_2, and is a dull, soft sound best heard at the apex.

Heart murmurs that are innocent (or functional) in origin are common through childhood (often called *Still's murmur*). Most innocent murmurs have these characteristics: soft, relatively short, systolic ejection murmur; medium pitch; vibratory; and best heard at the left lower sternal or midsternal border, with no radiation to the apex, base, or back.

Pregnant Women

The vital signs usually reveal that the resting pulse rate is increased by 10 to 15 beats per minute and that blood pressure is lower than the normal prepregnancy level. Blood pressure decreases to its lowest point during the second trimester and then slowly rises during the third trimester. Blood pressure varies with position. It is usually lowest in the left lateral recumbent position, a bit higher when supine (except for some who experience hypotension when supine), and highest when sitting.

Suspect pregnancy-induced hypertension with a sustained rise of 30 mm Hg systolic or 15 mm Hg diastolic under basal conditions.

Normal Range of Findings	Abnormal Findings

Palpation of the apical impulse is higher and lateral as compared with the normal position, because the enlarging uterus elevates the diaphragm and displaces the heart up and to the left and rotates it on its long axis.

Auscultation of the heart sounds reveals changes caused by the increased blood volume and workload:

Heart sounds
- Exaggerated splitting of S_1 and increased loudness of S_1
- A loud, easily heard S_3

Heart murmurs
- A systolic murmur in 90%, which disappears soon after delivery
- A continuous murmur arising from breast vasculature in 10%, the mammary souffle (pronounced *soof' f'l*).

Murmurs of aortic valve disease cannot be obliterated.

Older Adults

A gradual rise in systolic blood pressure is common in older patients; the diastolic blood pressure stays fairly constant, with a resulting widening of pulse pressure. Some older adults experience **orthostatic hypotension,** a sudden drop in blood pressure when rising to sit or stand.

The chest often increases in anteroposterior diameter in older patients. This makes it more difficult to palpate the apical impulse and to hear the splitting of S_2. The S_4 often occurs in older people with no known cardiac disease.

Occasional premature ectopic beats are common and do not necessarily indicate underlying heart disease. When in doubt, obtain an ECG; however, consider that the ECG records only 1 isolated minute and may need to be supplemented by 24-hour ambulatory heart monitoring.

The S_3 is associated with heart failure and is always abnormal when present after 40 years of age. (See Table 20.7, p. 530, in Jarvis: *Physical Examination and Health Assessment,* 3rd Canadian edition.)

Summary Checklist: Heart and Neck Vessels Examination

Neck
1. **Carotid pulse:** observe and palpate
2. **Jugular venous pulse:** observe
3. **Jugular venous pressure:** estimate

Precordium
1. **Inspection and palpation:**
   Describe location of apical impulse
   Note any heave (lift) or thrill
2. **Auscultation:**
   Identify anatomical areas where you listen
   Note rate and rhythm of heartbeat

Identify S_1 and S_2, and note any variation
Listen in systole and diastole for any extra heart sounds
Listen in systole and diastole for any murmurs
Repeat sequence with bell of stethoscope
Listen at apex with patient in left lateral position
Listen at base with patient in sitting position
3. **Engage in health promotion and teaching**

ABNORMAL FINDINGS

TABLE 12.1	Diastolic Extra Sounds

Third Heart Sound

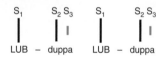

The S_3 is a ventricular filling sound. It occurs in early diastole during the rapid filling phase. Your hearing quickly accommodates to the S_3, so it is best heard when you listen initially. It sounds after S_2, is a dull soft sound, and is low-pitched, like "distant thunder." It is heard best in a quiet room, at the apex, with the bell held lightly (just enough to form a seal), and with the patient in the left lateral position.

The S_3 can be confused with a split S_2. Use these guidelines to distinguish the S_3:

- *Location:* The S_3 is heard at the apex or lower left sternal border; the split S_2 at the base.
- *Respiratory variation:* The S_3 does not vary in timing with respirations; the split S_2 does.
- *Pitch:* The S_3 is lower pitched; the pitch of the split S_2 stays the same.

The S_3 may be normal (physiological) or abnormal (pathological). The *physiological S_3* is heard frequently in children and young adults; it occasionally may persist after age 40 years, especially in women. The normal S_3 usually disappears when the patient sits up.

In adults, the S_3 is usually abnormal. The *pathological S_3* is also called a *ventricular gallop* or an S_3 *gallop*, and it persists when sitting up. The S_3 indicates decreased compliance of the ventricles, as in heart failure. The S_3 may be the earliest sign of heart failure.

The S_3 is also found in high cardiac output states in the absence of heart disease, such as hyperthyroidism, anemia, and pregnancy. When the primary conduction is corrected, the gallop disappears.

TABLE 12.1   Diastolic Extra Sounds—cont'd

Fourth Heart Sound

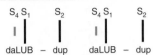

The **S₄** is a ventricular filling sound. It occurs when the atria contract late in diastole. It is heard immediately before **S₁**. This is a very soft sound, of very low pitch. You need a good bell, and you must listen for it. It is heard best at the apex, with the patient in the left lateral position.

A *physiological S₄* may occur in adults older than 40 or 50 years with no evidence of cardiovascular disease, especially after exercise.

A *pathological S₄* is termed an *atrial gallop* or an *S₄ gallop*. It occurs with decreased compliance of the ventricle, such as in coronary artery disease and cardiomyopathy, and with systolic overload (afterload), including outflow obstruction to the ventricle (aortic stenosis), and systemic hypertension. A left-sided S₄ occurs with these conditions. It is heard best at the apex, in the left lateral position.

A right-sided S₄ is less common. It is heard at the left lower sternal border and may increase with inspiration. It occurs with pulmonary stenosis or pulmonary hypertension.

Pericardial Friction Rub

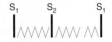

Inflammation of the pericardium gives rise to a friction rub. The sound is high pitched and scratchy, like sandpaper being rubbed. It is best heard with the diaphragm of the stethoscope, with the patient sitting up and leaning forward, and with the breath held in expiration.

A friction rub can be heard any place on the precordium, but is usually best heard at the apex and left lower sternal border, places where the pericardium comes in close contact with the chest wall. Timing may be systolic and diastolic.

The friction rub of pericarditis is common during the first week after a myocardial infarction and may last only a few hours.

TABLE 12.2	Abnormal Pulsations on the Precordium

Base

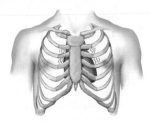

Base

A *thrill* in the second and third right interspaces occurs with severe aortic stenosis and systemic hypertension.

A thrill in the second and third left interspaces occurs with pulmonic stenosis and pulmonic hypertension.

Left Sternal Border

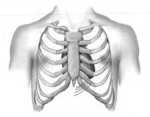

Left Sternal Border

A *lift (heave)* occurs with right ventricular hypertrophy, as found in pulmonic valve disease, pulmonic hypertension, and chronic lung disease. You feel a diffuse lifting impulse during systole at the left lower sternal border. It may be associated with retraction at the apex because the left ventricle is rotated posteriorly by the enlarged right ventricle.

Apex

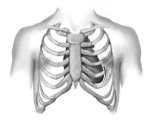

Apex

Cardiac enlargement displaces the apical impulse laterally and over a wider area when left ventricular hypertrophy and dilation are present. This is *volume overload,* as in mitral regurgitation, aortic regurgitation, and left-to-right shunts.

Apex

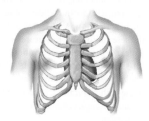

Apex

The apical impulse is increased in force and duration, but is not necessarily displaced to the left when left ventricular hypertrophy occurs alone without dilation. This is *pressure overload,* as found in aortic stenosis or systemic hypertension.

Images © Pat Thomas, 2006.

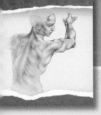

CHAPTER 13

Peripheral Vascular System and Lymphatic System

STRUCTURE AND FUNCTION

The vascular system consists of the vessels in the body. Vessels are tubes for transporting fluid, such as blood or lymph.

The heart pumps freshly oxygenated blood and nutrients through the arteries to all body tissues. The major artery to the leg is the **femoral artery**, which passes under the inguinal ligament (Fig. 13.1).

Veins drain the deoxygenated blood and its waste products from the tissues and return it to the heart (Fig. 13.2).

The lymphatics form a completely separate vessel system, which retrieves excess fluid and plasma proteins from the tissue spaces and returns them to the bloodstream. The lymphatic system also forms a major part of the

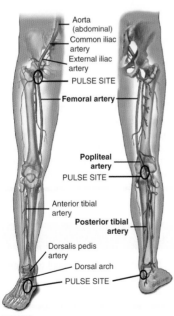

13.1 Arteries in the leg. (© Pat Thomas, 2010.)

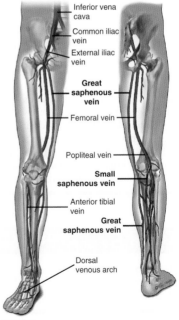

13.2 Veins in the leg. (© Pat Thomas, 2010.)

157

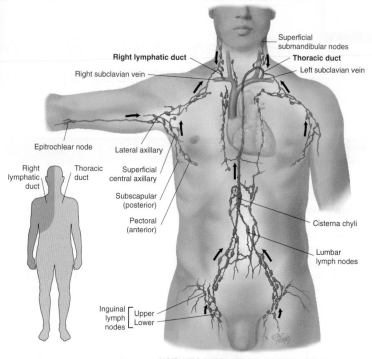

LYMPHATIC DUCTS AND DRAINAGE PATTERNS

13.3 *(© Pat Thomas, 2010.)*

immune system that defends the body against disease.

Cervical lymph nodes drain the head and neck and are described in Chapter 6. **Axillary** lymph nodes drain the breast and upper arm and are described in Chapter 10.

The **epitrochlear** lymph node is in the antecubital fossa and drains the hand and lower arm (Fig. 13.3). The **inguinal** nodes in the groin drain most of the lymph of the lower extremity, the external genitalia, and the anterior abdominal wall.

SUBJECTIVE DATA

1. Leg pain or cramps
2. Skin changes on arms or legs
3. Swelling in the arms or legs
4. Lymph node enlargement (swollen glands)
5. Medications

OBJECTIVE DATA

PREPARATION

During a complete physical examination, examine the arms at the very beginning when you are checking the vital signs and the patient is sitting. Examine the legs directly after the abdominal examination, while the patient is still supine. Then have the patient stand up to evaluate the leg veins.

EQUIPMENT NEEDED (OCCASIONALLY)

Paper tape measure
Tourniquet or blood pressure cuff
Stethoscope
Doppler ultrasonic stethoscope

Normal Range of Findings	Abnormal Findings
Inspect and Palpate the Arms	
Note colour of skin and nail beds; temperature, texture, and turgor of skin; and the presence of any lesions, edema, or clubbing, as described in Chapter 5.	
With the patient's hands near the level of his or her heart, check **capillary refill.** Depress and blanch the nail beds; release and note the time for colour return. Usually, the vessels refill within a fraction of a second. Consider it normal if the colour returns in less than 1 or 2 seconds. Note conditions that can skew your findings, including a cool room, decreased body temperature, cigarette smoking, peripheral edema, and anemia.	Refill time of more than 1 or 2 seconds signifies vasoconstriction or decreased cardiac output (hypovolemia, heart failure, shock). The hands are cold, clammy, and pale.
The two arms should be symmetrical in size.	Edema of upper extremities occurs when lymphatic drainage is obstructed, which may occur after breast surgery. (See Table 21.2, p. 560, in Jarvis: *Physical Examination and Health Assessment,* 3rd Canadian edition.)
Note the presence of any scars on hands and arms. Many occur normally with usual childhood abrasions or with occupations involving hand tools.	Needle tracks in antecubital fossae occur with intravenous drug use; linear scars in wrists may signify past self-inflicted injury.

Continued

Normal Range of Findings	Abnormal Findings
Palpate both radial pulses, noting rate, rhythm, elasticity of vessel wall, and equal force. Grade the force (amplitude) on a four-point scale:	The pulse is full and bounding (3+) in hyperkinetic states (exercise, anxiety, fever), anemia, and hyperthyroidism.
3+: increased, full, bounding	The pulse is weak and "thready" in shock and peripheral arterial disease. (See Table 13.1, for illustrations of these and irregular pulse rhythms.)
2+: **normal**	
1+: weak	
0: absent	
Palpate the brachial pulses; their force should be equal bilaterally.	
Check the epitrochlear lymph nodes in the depression above and behind the medial condyle of the humerus. This node is normally not palpable.	An enlarged epitrochlear node occurs with infection of the hand or forearm.
	Epitrochlear nodes are palpable in conditions of generalized lymphadenopathy: lymphoma, chronic lymphocytic leukemia, sarcoidosis, infections, and mononucleosis.

Inspect and Palpate the Legs

Normal Range of Findings	Abnormal Findings
Inspect both legs together, noting skin colour, hair distribution, venous pattern, size (swelling or atrophy), and any skin lesions or ulcers.	Abnormalities include pallor with vasoconstriction, erythema with vasodilation, and cyanosis.
	Leg ulcers occur with chronic arterial and chronic venous disease. (See Table 21.4, p. 562, in Jarvis: *Physical Examination and Health Assessment,* 3rd Canadian edition.)
Hair normally covers the legs. Even if leg hair is shaved, you will still note hair on the dorsa of the toes.	In malnutrition, skin is thin, shiny, and atrophic; nails have thick ridges; hair loss occurs; and ulcers and gangrene may be present. Malnutrition, pallor, and coolness occur with arterial insufficiency.
The venous pattern is normally flat and barely visible. Note obvious varicosities, although these are best assessed while the patient is standing.	
Both legs should be symmetrical in size without swelling or atrophy. If the lower legs appear asymmetrical or if deep vein thrombosis (DVT) is suspected, measure the calf circumference with a nonstretchable tape measure. Measure at the widest point, in exactly the same place on both legs, the same number of centimetres down from the patella or other landmark. Record your findings in centimetres.	Diffuse bilateral edema occurs with systemic illnesses.
	Acute, unilateral, painful swelling and asymmetry of calves of 1 cm or more is abnormal; refer the patient to determine whether DVT is present.
	Asymmetry of 1 to 3 cm occurs with mild lymphedema; 3 to 5 cm with moderate lymphedema; and greater than 5 cm with severe lymphedema. (See Table 21.2, p. 560, in Jarvis: *Physical Examination & Health Assessment,* 3rd Canadian edition.)

Normal Range of Findings	Abnormal Findings
Palpate for temperature (using the dorsa of your hand) along the legs and down to the feet, comparing symmetrical spots. The skin should be warm and equal bilaterally. Both feet may be cool because of environmental factors, such as cool room temperature, apprehension, and cigarette smoking. If there is any increase in temperature higher up the leg, note whether it is gradual or abrupt.	With arterial deficit, one foot or leg may be cool or the temperature may drop suddenly as you move down the leg.
Palpate the inguinal lymph nodes. It is not unusual to find palpable nodes that are small (1 cm or less), movable, and nontender.	Nodes are not normally enlarged, tender or fixed in area.
Palpate these peripheral arteries in both legs: femoral, popliteal, posterior tibial, and dorsalis pedis. Grade the force on the four-point scale.	
Femoral Pulse. Locate the **femoral arteries** just below the inguinal ligament, halfway between the pubis and anterior superior iliac spines (see Fig. 13.1). To help expose the femoral area, particularly in obese patients, ask the patient to bend his or her knees to the side in a froglike position. Press firmly and then slowly release, noting the pulse tap under your fingertips. If this pulse is weak or diminished, auscultate the site for a bruit.	A bruit occurs with turbulent blood flow, indicating partial occlusion.
Popliteal Pulse. This is a more diffuse pulse and can be difficult to localize. With the patient's leg extended but relaxed, anchor your thumbs on the knee, and curl your fingers around into the popliteal fossa. Press your fingers forward hard to compress the artery against the bone. The pulse is often just lateral to the medial tendon. A normal popliteal pulse is often impossible to palpate.	
Posterior Tibial Pulse. Curve your fingers around the medial malleolus (Fig. 13.4). You will feel the tapping right behind it in the groove between the malleolus and the Achilles tendon.	

Continued

Normal Range of Findings	Abnormal Findings

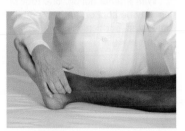

13.4 Posterior tibial pulse.

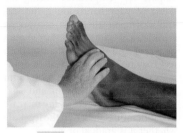

13.5 Dorsalis pedis pulse.

Dorsalis Pedis Pulse. This requires a very light touch. It is normally just lateral to and parallel with the extensor tendon of the big toe (Fig. 13.5).

Check for pretibial edema. Firmly depress the skin over the tibia or the medial malleolus for 5 seconds and release. Your finger should normally leave no indentation, although a pit is commonly seen if the patient has been standing all day or is pregnant.

Bilateral, dependent, pitting edema occurs with heart failure, diabetic neuropathy, and hepatic cirrhosis.

If pitting edema is present, grade it on this scale:

1+: Mild pitting, slight indentation, no perceptible swelling of the leg
2+: Moderate pitting, indentation that subsides rapidly
3+: Deep pitting, indentation that remains for a short time, swelling of leg
4+: Very deep pitting, indentation lasts a long time, gross swelling and distortion of leg

Unilateral edema occurs with occlusion of a deep vein and unilaterally or bilaterally with lymphatic obstruction. With these factors, it is "brawny" or nonpitting and feels hard to the touch.

This scale is subjective. Because peripheral edema is a common clinical sign in a great number of conditions, it is important to detect true changes in the most accurate way available. Check with your own institution to conform to a consistently used scale.

Ask the patient to stand so you can assess the venous system. Note any visible, dilated, or tortuous veins. If varicose veins are present, ask if they cause pain, swelling, fatigue, or cramping.

Varicosities occur in the saphenous veins. (See Table 21.5, p. 563, in Jarvis: *Physical Examination and Health Assessment,* 3rd Canadian edition.)

Normal Range of Findings	Abnormal Findings

Additional Techniques

The Doppler Ultrasonic Stethoscope. Use this device to detect a weak peripheral pulse, to monitor blood pressure in infants and children, and to measure a low blood pressure or blood pressure in a lower extremity (Fig. 13.6). The Doppler ultrasonic stethoscope magnifies pulsatile sounds from the heart and blood vessels. Place a drop of coupling gel on the end of the handheld transducer. Place the transducer over a pulse site, swivelled at a 45-degree angle. Apply very light pressure; locate the pulse site by the swishing, whooshing sound.

 DEVELOPMENTAL CONSIDERATIONS

Infants and Children

Transient acrocyanosis (i.e., symmetrical cyanosis of the hands and wrists, feet and ankles) and skin mottling may occur at birth. Pulse force should be normal and symmetrical. Pulse force should also be the same in the upper and lower extremities.

Weak pulses occur with vasoconstriction or diminished cardiac output.

Full, bounding pulses occur with patent ductus arteriosus as a result of the large left-to-right shunt.

Diminished or absent femoral pulses in the presence of normal upper extremity pulses are suggestive of coarctation of aorta.

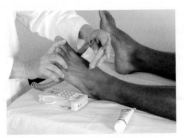

13.6 Using the Doppler to locate a pulse.

Continued

Normal Range of Findings	Abnormal Findings
Lymph nodes are often palpable in healthy infants and children. They are small, firm (shotty), mobile, and non-tender. Their palpability may be the sequelae of past infection, such as diaper rash (inguinal nodes), or a respiratory infection (cervical nodes). Vaccinations can also produce local lymphadenopathy. Note characteristics of any palpable nodes and whether they are local or generalized.	Enlarged, warm, tender nodes indicate current infection. Look for source of infection.

Pregnant Women

Expect diffuse, bilateral, pitting edema in the lower extremities, especially at the end of the day and into the third trimester. Varicose veins in the legs are also common in the third trimester.	Remain alert for generalized edema in addition to hypertension, which are suggestive of preeclampsia, a dangerous obstetric condition.

Older Adults

The dorsalis pedis and posterior tibial pulses may become more difficult to find. Trophic changes associated with arterial insufficiency (thin, shiny skin; thick-ridged nails; loss of hair on lower legs) also occur normally with aging.

Summary Checklist: Peripheral Vascular Examination

1. **Inspect arms** for colour, size, and any lesions
2. **Palpate pulses** (radial, brachial)
3. **Check epitrochlear node**
4. **Inspect legs** for colour, size, any lesions, and trophic skin changes
5. **Palpate the skin for temperature** of feet and legs
6. **Palpate inguinal nodes**
7. **Palpate pulses in lower extremities** (femoral, popliteal, posterior tibial, dorsalis pedis)
8. **Engage in health promotion and teaching**

ABNORMAL FINDINGS

TABLE 13.1	Variations in Arterial Pulse

Description	Associated With
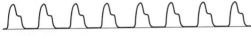 ***Weak "Thready" Pulse: 1+*** Hard to palpate, hard to find, may fade in and out, easily obliterated by pressure.	Decreased cardiac output; peripheral arterial disease; aortic valve stenosis.
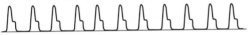 ***Full, Bounding Pulse: 3+*** Easily palpable, pounds under examiner's fingertips.	Hyperkinetic states (exercise, anxiety, fever), anemia, hyperthyroidism.
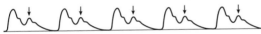 ***Water–Hammer (Corrigan's) Pulse: 3+*** Greater than normal force, then sudden collapse.	Aortic valve regurgitation; patent ductus arteriosus.
Pulsus Bigeminus Coupled rhythm, wherein every other beat comes early, or normal beat followed by premature beat. Force of premature beat is decreased because of shortened cardiac filling time.	Conduction disturbance (e.g., premature ventricular contraction, premature atrial contraction).
Pulsus Alternans Rhythm is regular, but force varies with alternating beats of large and small amplitude.	When heart rate is normal, pulsus alternans occurs with severe left ventricular failure, which in turn is due to ischemic heart disease, valvular heart disease, chronic hypertension, or cardiomyopathy.

Continued

TABLE 13.1	Variations in Arterial Pulse—cont'd
Description	**Associated With**

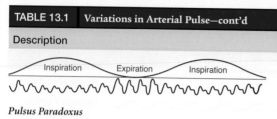

Pulsus Paradoxus

Amplitude of beats: weaker with inspiration, stronger with expiration. Rhythm best determined during blood pressure measurement; reading decreases (>10 mm Hg) during inspiration and increases with expiration.

A common finding in cardiac tamponade (pericardial effusion in which high pressure compresses the heart and blocks cardiac output); also in severe bronchospasm of acute asthma.

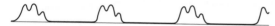

Pulsus Bisferiens

Two strong systolic peaks, with a dip in between in each pulse; best assessed at the carotid artery.

Aortic valve stenosis plus regurgitation.

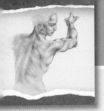

CHAPTER 14

The Abdomen

STRUCTURE AND FUNCTION

The **abdomen** is a large oval cavity extending from the diaphragm down to the top of the pelvis (Fig. 14.1). For convenience in description, the abdominal wall is divided into four quadrants by imaginary vertical and horizontal lines bisecting the umbilicus.

The **aorta** is just to the left of midline in the upper abdomen (Fig. 14.2). It descends behind the peritoneum, and at 2 cm below the umbilicus, it bifurcates into the right and left common iliac arteries opposite the fourth lumbar vertebra.

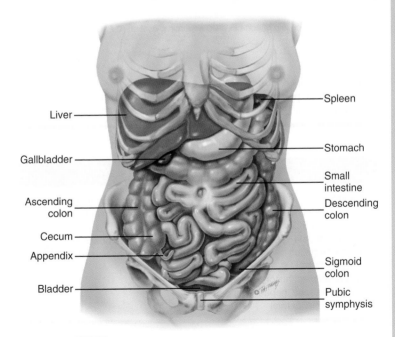

Liver
Gallbladder
Ascending colon
Cecum
Appendix
Bladder

Spleen
Stomach
Small intestine
Descending colon
Sigmoid colon
Pubic symphysis

14.1 Position of abdominal organs. (© Pat Thomas, 2006.)

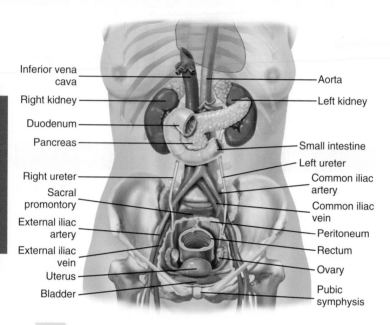

14.2 Relationship of aorta to deep abdominal viscera. *(© Pat Thomas, 2006.)*

The bean-shaped **kidneys** are retroperitoneal, or posterior to the abdominal contents. The **spleen** is a soft mass of lymphatic tissue on the posterolateral wall of the abdomen, immediately under the diaphragm.

SUBJECTIVE DATA

1. Appetite
2. Dysphagia (difficulty swallowing)
3. Food intolerance
4. Abdominal pain
5. Nausea/vomiting
6. Bowel habits
7. Past abdominal history (ulcer, gallbladder disease, hepatitis, appendicitis, colitis, hernia)
8. Medications (prescription, over-the-counter [including antacids], supplements)
9. Alcohol and tobacco
10. Nutritional assessment (24-hour recall)

OBJECTIVE DATA

PREPARATION

Turn on a strong overhead light and a secondary stand light. Expose the patient's abdomen so that it is fully visible. Drape the genitalia and female breasts.

The following measures will enhance abdominal wall relaxation:

- Have the patient empty his or her bladder, saving a urine specimen if needed.
- Keep the room warm.
- Position the patient supine, with the head on a pillow, knees bent or on a pillow, and the arms at the sides or across the chest.
- Keep the stethoscope endpiece and your hands warm, and your fingernails very short.
- Examine any painful areas last to avoid muscle guarding.
- Use distraction: breathing exercises; emotive imagery; your low, soothing voice; and the person relating his or her abdominal history while you palpate.

EQUIPMENT NEEDED

Small ruler marked in centimeters
Skin-marking pen
Alcohol wipe (to clean endpiece)
Drape
Stethoscope

Normal Range of Findings	Abnormal Findings
Inspect the Abdomen	
Contour. Stand on the patient's right side and stoop or sit to gaze across the abdomen. Determine the profile from the rib margin to the pubic bone, normally flat to rounded. A scaphoid abdomen caves in.	Protuberant abdomen, abdominal distension are abnormal (see Table 14.1).
Symmetry. Shine a light across the abdomen toward you, or shine it lengthwise across the patient. The abdomen should be symmetrical bilaterally. Note any localized bulging, visible mass, or asymmetry.	Bulges, masses. Hernia: protrusion of abdominal viscera through abnormal opening in muscle wall. (See Table 22.4, p. 601, in Jarvis: *Physical Examination and Health Assessment,* 3rd Canadian edition.)

Continued

Normal Range of Findings	Abnormal Findings
Umbilicus. It is normally midline and inverted with no sign of discoloration, inflammation, or hernia. It becomes everted and pushed upward during pregnancy.	Everted with ascites or underlying mass. Deeply sunken with obesity. Enlarged and everted with umbilical hernia. Bluish periumbilical colour: with intra-abdominal bleeding (Cullen's sign), although rare. Redness with localized inflammation. Jaundice with hepatitis (shows best in natural daylight).
Skin. The surface is smooth and even, with homogeneous colour. There are normally no lesions, although sometimes well-healed surgical scars are present. If a scar is present, draw its location in the patient's record, indicating the length in centimetres.	Skin glistening and taut with ascites. Cutaneous angiomas (spider nevi) occur with portal hypertension or liver disease. Lesions, rashes (see Chapter 5).
Pulsation or Movement. Pulsations from the aorta may show beneath the skin in the epigastric area, particularly in thin patients with good muscle wall relaxation. Respiratory movement also shows in the abdomen, particularly in men.	Marked pulsation of the aorta with widened pulse pressure (e.g., hypertension, aortic insufficiency, thyrotoxicosis), and aortic aneurysm. Markedly visible peristalsis, together with a distended abdomen, indicates intestinal obstruction.
Demeanour. A comfortable patient is relaxed quietly on the examining table and has a benign facial expression and slow, even respirations.	Restlessness and constant turning to find comfort occur with the colicky pain of gastroenteritis or bowel obstruction. Absolute stillness, resisting any movement, occurs with the pain of peritonitis. Upward flexing of the knees, facial grimacing, and rapid, uneven respirations also indicate pain.

Auscultate Bowel Sounds and Vascular Sounds

Auscultation is done next because percussion and palpation can increase peristalsis, which would give a false interpretation of bowel sounds. Use the diaphragm end piece and hold the stethoscope lightly against the skin. Begin in the right lower quadrant (RLQ) at the ileocecal valve area because bowel sounds are normally always present here.

Normal Range of Findings	Abnormal Findings

Bowel Sounds. Note the character and frequency: normally high-pitched, gurgling, cascading sounds, occurring irregularly anywhere from 5 to 30 times per minute. Do not bother to count them. Judge if they are normal, hypoactive, or hyperactive.

Abnormal bowel sounds have two distinct patterns:
1. Hyperactive sounds are loud, high-pitched, rushing, tinkling sounds that signal increased motility, and may indicate bowel obstruction.
2. Hypoactive or absent sounds may occur after abdominal surgery or with inflammation of the peritoneum. (See Table 22.5, p. 603, in Jarvis: *Physical Examination and Health Assessment,* 3rd Canadian edition.)

Vascular Sounds. Using firmer pressure and the bell of the stethoscope, listen over the aorta, renal arteries, iliac, and femoral arteries, especially in patients with hypertension (Fig. 14.3). Note the presence of any vascular sounds or **bruits.** Usually, no such sound is present.

Note location, pitch, and timing of a vascular sound.

A systolic bruit is a pulsatile, blowing sound and occurs with occlusion of an artery.

Venous hum and peritoneal friction rub are rare. (See Table 22.6, p. 603, in Jarvis: *Physical Examination and Health Assessment,* 3rd Canadian edition.)

Percuss General Tympany, Liver Span, and Splenic Dullness

General Tympany. Percuss lightly in all four quadrants. Tympany should predominate because air in the intestines rises to the surface when the patient is supine.

Dullness occurs over a solid structure (e.g., liver), a distended bladder, adipose tissue, fluid, or a mass.

Hyperresonance is present with gaseous distension.

Continued

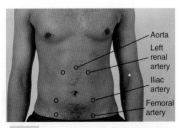

14.3 Sites to listen for vascular sounds.

Aorta
Left renal artery
Iliac artery
Femoral artery

Normal Range of Findings	Abnormal Findings

Liver Span. Measure the height of the liver in the right midclavicular line. Begin in the area of lung resonance and percuss down the intercostal spaces until the sound changes to a dull quality. Mark the spot, usually in the fifth intercostal space. Then find abdominal tympany and percuss up in the midclavicular line. Mark where the sound changes from tympany to a dull sound, normally at the right costal margin.

Elongation of the liver span indicates liver enlargement (hepatomegaly).

Detection of liver borders is rendered inaccurate by dullness above fifth intercostal space, which occurs with lung disease (e.g., pleural effusion or consolidation). Detection at the lower border is rendered inaccurate when dullness is pushed up with ascites, pregnancy, or with gas distension in colon, which obscures lower border.

Measure the distance between the two marks; the normal liver span in adults ranges from 6 to 12 cm (Fig. 14.4). Taller people have longer livers. Men also have a larger liver span than do women of the same height. Overall, the mean liver span is 10.5 cm in men and 7 cm in women.

Splenic Dullness. Locate the spleen by percussing for a dull note from the ninth to the eleventh intercostal spaces just behind the left midaxillary line. The area of splenic dullness is normally not wider than 7 cm in adults and should not encroach on the normal tympany over the gastric air bubble.

A dull note forward of the midaxillary line indicates enlargement of the spleen, as occurs with mononucleosis, trauma, and infection.

Palpate Surface and Deep Areas, Liver Edge, Spleen, and Kidneys

Light and Deep Palpation. Begin with **light palpation**. With the first four fingers close together, depress the skin about 1 cm. Make a gentle rotary motion, lift the fingers (do not drag them), and move clockwise.

Muscle guarding.
Rigidity.
Large masses.
Tenderness.

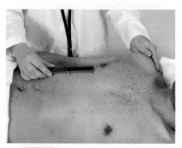

14.4 Measuring the liver span.

Normal Range of Findings	Abnormal Findings

As you circle the abdomen, discriminate between voluntary muscle guarding and involuntary rigidity. **Voluntary guarding** occurs when the patient is cold, tense, or ticklish. It is bilateral, and the muscles relax slightly during exhalation. Use relaxation measures to try to eliminate this type of guarding, or it will interfere with deep palpation. If rigidity persists, it is probably involuntary.

Involuntary rigidity is a constant, boardlike hardness of the muscles. It is a protective mechanism accompanying acute inflammation of the peritoneum. It may be unilateral, and the same area usually becomes painful when the patient increases intra-abdominal pressure by attempting a sit-up.

Now perform **deep palpation**, pushing down about 5 to 8 cm. Moving clockwise, explore the entire abdomen.

To overcome the resistance of a very large or obese abdomen, use a bimanual technique. Place your two hands on top of each other. The top hand does the pushing; the bottom hand is relaxed and can concentrate on the sense of palpation. With either technique, note the location, size, consistency, and mobility of any palpable organs, and the presence of any abnormal enlargement, tenderness, or masses. Remember that some structures are normally palpable, as illustrated in Fig. 14.5.

Mild tenderness normally is present when palpating the sigmoid colon. Any other tenderness should be investigated.

Tenderness occurs with local inflammation, with inflammation of the peritoneum or underlying organ, and with an enlarged organ whose capsule is stretched.

If you identify a mass, first distinguish it from a normally palpable structure or an enlarged organ. Then note the following:

1. Location
2. Size
3. Shape
4. Consistency (soft, firm, hard)
5. Surface (smooth, nodular)
6. Mobility (including movement with respirations)
7. Pulsatility
8. Tenderness

Continued

Normal Range of Findings	Abnormal Findings

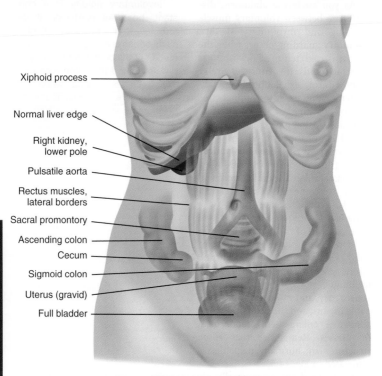

Xiphoid process

Normal liver edge

Right kidney, lower pole

Pulsatile aorta

Rectus muscles, lateral borders

Sacral promontory

Ascending colon

Cecum

Sigmoid colon

Uterus (gravid)

Full bladder

NORMALLY PALPABLE STRUCTURES

14.5 Normally palpable abdominal structures. *(© Pat Thomas, 2006.)*

Liver. Place your left hand under the patient's back, parallel to the eleventh and twelfth ribs, and lift up to support the abdominal contents. Place your right hand on the right upper quadrant (RUQ), with fingers parallel to the midline (Fig. 14.6). Push deeply down and under the right costal margin. Ask the patient to take a deep breath. It is normal to feel the edge of the liver bump your fingertips as the diaphragm pushes it down during inhalation. It feels like a firm, regular ridge. The liver is often not palpable, and you may feel nothing firm.

Except with a depressed diaphragm, a liver palpated more than 1 to 2 cm below the right costal margin is enlarged. Record the number of centimetres it descends, and note its consistency (hard, nodular) and any tenderness.

Normal Range of Findings	Abnormal Findings

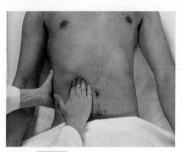

14.6 Palpating the liver.

Spleen. Normally, the spleen is not palpable and must be enlarged three times its normal size to be felt.

Reach your left hand over the abdomen and behind the left side at the eleventh and twelfth ribs. Lift up for support. Place your right hand obliquely on the left upper quadrant (LUQ) with the fingers pointing toward the left axilla and just inferior to the rib margin. Push your hand deeply down and under the left costal margin, and ask the patient to take a deep breath. You should feel nothing firm. When enlarged, the spleen slides out and bumps your fingertips.

Kidneys. Search for the right kidney by placing your hands together in a "duck bill" position at the patient's right flank. Press your two hands together firmly, and ask the patient to take a deep breath. With most people, you will feel no change. Occasionally, you may feel the lower pole of the right kidney as a round, smooth mass slide between your fingers. Either condition is normal.

CRITICAL FINDING: The spleen enlarges with mononucleosis and trauma. (See Table 22.7, p. 605, in Jarvis: *Physical Examination and Health Assessment,* 3rd Canadian edition.) If you feel enlargement of the spleen, refer the patient; *do not continue to palpate.* An enlarged spleen is friable and can rupture easily with overpalpation.

Describe the number of centimetres it extends below the left costal margin.

Enlarged kidney.
Kidney mass.

Continued

Normal Range of Findings	Abnormal Findings

The left kidney sits 1 cm higher than the right kidney and is not normally palpable.

Aorta. Using your opposing thumb and fingers, palpate the aortic pulsation in the upper abdomen slightly to the left of midline. It is normally 2.5 to 4 cm wide in adults, and pulsates in an anterior direction.

Widened aorta with aneurysm.

Prominent lateral pulsation with aortic aneurysm. (See Tables 22.6 and 22.7, pages 603–604, in Jarvis: *Physical Examination and Health Assessment*, 3rd Canadian edition.)

CRITICAL FINDING: If a bruit is heard on auscultation, you should *not* palpate the area, to avoid rupturing an aortic aneurysm. Report findings immediately.

Sharp pain occurs with inflammation of the kidney or paranephric area.

Costovertebral Angle Tenderness. Place one hand over the twelfth rib at the costovertebral angle on the back. Thump that hand with the ulnar edge of your other fist. The patient normally feels a thud but no pain.

Special Procedures

Rebound Tenderness (Blumberg's Sign). Choose a site away from the painful area. Hold your hand 90 degrees, or perpendicular, to the abdomen. Push down slowly and deeply, then lift up *quickly*. This makes structures that are indented by palpation rebound suddenly. A normal, or negative, response is absence of pain on release of pressure. Perform this test at the end of the examination because it can cause severe pain and muscle rigidity.

Pain on release of pressure confirms rebound tenderness, which is a reliable sign of peritoneal inflammation. Peritoneal inflammation accompanies appendicitis.

Cough tenderness localized to a specific spot also signals peritoneal irritation. Refer the patient with suspected appendicitis for computed tomographic scanning.

Normal Range of Findings	Abnormal Findings

Inspiratory Arrest (Murphy's Sign). Normally, palpating the liver causes no pain. In a patient with inflammation of the gallbladder, or cholecystitis, pain occurs. Hold your fingers under the liver border. Ask the patient to take a deep breath. A normal response is to complete the deep breath without pain.

When the test result is positive, as the descending liver pushes the inflamed gallbladder onto the examining hand, the patient feels sharp pain and abruptly stops inspiration midway. (Note: This sign is less accurate in patients older than 60 years of age, who may not have any abdominal tenderness.)

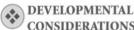 **DEVELOPMENTAL CONSIDERATIONS**

The Infant

The contour of the abdomen is protuberant because of the immature abdominal musculature. The skin contains a fine, superficial venous pattern. This may be visible in lightly pigmented children until puberty.

Scaphoid shape occurs with dehydration.
Dilated veins.

The abdomen shows respiratory movement. The only other abdominal movement is occasional peristalsis, which may be visible because of the thin musculature.

Marked peristalsis occurs with pyloric stenosis.

Auscultation yields only bowel sounds, the metallic tinkling of peristalsis. There should be no vascular sounds.

Bruit.
Venous hum.

Children

In children younger than age 4 years, the abdomen looks protuberant when the child is both supine and standing. After age 4 years, the potbelly remains when standing because of lumbar lordosis, but the abdomen looks flat when supine. Normal movement on the abdomen includes respirations, which remain abdominal until 7 years of age.

A scaphoid abdomen is associated with dehydration or malnutrition.
Before 7 years of age, abdominal respirations are absent with inflammation of the peritoneum.

Continued

Normal Range of Findings	Abnormal Findings

Older Adults

On inspection, you may note increased deposits of subcutaneous fat on the abdomen and hips because it is redistributed away from the extremities. The abdominal musculature is thinner and has less tone than that of the younger adult, so in the absence of obesity you may note peristalsis.

Because of the thinner, softer abdominal wall, the organs may be easier to palpate (in the absence of obesity). The liver is easier to palpate. Normally, you will feel the liver edge at or just below the costal margin. With distended lungs and a depressed diaphragm, the liver is palpated lower, descending 1–2 cm below the costal margin with inhalation. The kidneys are easier to palpate.

Abdominal rigidity with acute abdominal conditions is less common in older adults.

Older adults with conditions that cause severe abdominal pain ("acute abdomen") often complain of less pain than do younger patients.

Summary Checklist: Abdomen Examination

1. **Inspection:**
   Contour
   Symmetry
   Umbilicus
   Skin
   Pulsation or movement
   Hair distribution
   Demeanour
2. **Auscultation:**
   Bowel sounds
   Any vascular sounds
3. **Percussion:**
   All four quadrants
   Borders of liver, spleen
4. **Palpation:**
   Light palpation in all four quadrants
   Deeper palpation in all four quadrants
   Palpation for liver, spleen, and kidneys
5. **Engage in health promotion and teaching**

ABNORMAL FINDINGS

TABLE 14.1	Abdominal Distension

Obesity

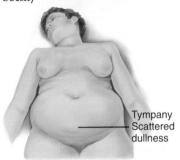

Tympany
Scattered
dullness

Inspection. Uniformly rounded. Umbilicus sunken (it adheres to peritoneum, and layers of fat are superficial to it).
Auscultation. Normal bowel sounds.
Percussion. Tympany. Scattered dullness over adipose tissue.
Palpation. Normal. May be hard to feel through thick abdominal wall.

Air or Gas

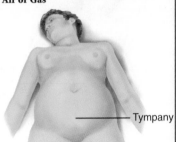

Tympany

Inspection. Single round curve.
Auscultation. Depends on cause of gas (e.g., decreased or absent bowel sounds with ileus); hyperactive with early intestinal obstruction.
Percussion. Tympany over large area.
Palpation. May have muscle spasm of abdominal wall.

Ascites

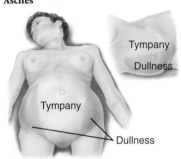

Tympany
Dullness
Tympany
Dullness

Inspection. Single curve. Everted umbilicus. Bulging flanks when supine. Taut, glistening skin, recent weight gain, increase in abdominal girth.
Auscultation. Normal bowel sounds over intestines. Diminished over ascitic fluid.
Percussion. Tympany at top where intestines float. Dull over fluid. Produces fluid wave and shifting dullness.
Palpation. Taut skin and increased intra-abdominal pressure limit palpation.

Ovarian Cyst (Large)

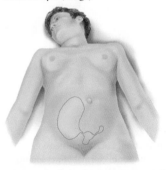

Inspection. Curve in lower half of abdomen, midline. Everted umbilicus.
Auscultation. Normal bowel sounds over upper abdomen where intestines pushed superiorly.
Percussion. Top dull over fluid. Intestines pushed superiorly. Large cyst produces fluid wave and shifting dullness.
Palpation. Aortic pulsation present (in ascites, it is not).

Continued

TABLE 14.1   Abdominal Distension—cont'd

Pregnancy*

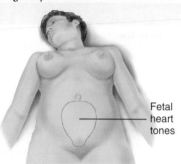

Fetal heart tones

Inspection. Single curve. Umbilicus protruding. Breasts engorged.
Auscultation. Fetal heart tones. Bowel sounds diminished.
Percussion. Tympany over intestines. Dull over enlarging uterus.
Palpation. Fetal parts. Fetal movements.

Feces

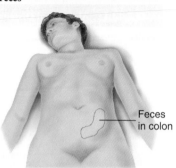

Feces in colon

Inspection. Localized distension.
Auscultation. Normal bowel sounds.
Percussion. Tympany predominates. Scattered dullness over fecal mass.
Palpation. Plastic-like or ropelike mass with feces in intestines.

Tumour

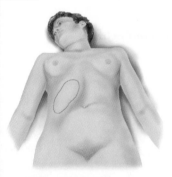

Inspection. Localized distension.
Auscultation. Normal bowel sounds.
Percussion. Dull over mass if reaches up to skin surface.
Palpation. Used to define borders and distinguish from enlarged organ or normally palpable structure.

*Obviously a normal finding, pregnancy is included for comparison of conditions causing abdominal distension.

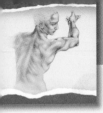

CHAPTER 15

Musculo-Skeletal System

STRUCTURE AND FUNCTION

The musculo-skeletal system consists of the body's bones, joints, and muscles.

A **joint** (or articulation) is the place of union of two or more bones. Joints are the functional units of the musculo-skeletal system because they enable the mobility needed for activities of daily living (ADLs).

Synovial joints are freely movable because they have bones that are separated from each other and that are enclosed in a joint cavity (Fig. 15.1). This cavity is filled with a lubricant called synovial fluid.

In synovial joints, a layer of resilient **cartilage** covers the surface of opposing bones. The cartilage cushions the bones and provides a smooth surface to facilitate movement. Each joint is surrounded by a fibrous capsule and is supported by ligaments. **Ligaments** are fibrous bands running directly from one bone to another that strengthen the joint and help prevent movement in undesirable directions. A **bursa** is an enclosed sac filled with viscous synovial fluid, much like a joint. **Bursae** are located in areas of potential friction (e.g., subacromial bursa of the shoulder, prepatellar bursa of the knee), and help muscles and tendons glide smoothly over bone.

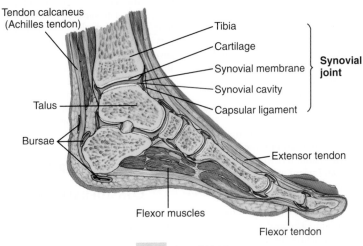

15.1 Synovial joints.

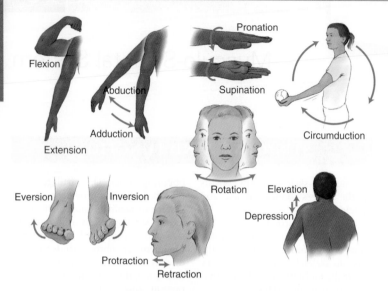

SKELETAL MUSCLE MOVEMENTS

15.2   *(© Pat Thomas, 2006.)*

Skeletal **muscle** is attached to bone by a **tendon,** a strong fibrous cord. Skeletal muscles produce the following movements (Fig. 15.2):

1. Flexion: bending a limb at a joint
2. Extension: straightening a limb at a joint
3. Abduction: moving a limb away from the midline of the body
4. Adduction: moving a limb toward the midline of the body
5. Pronation: turning the forearm so the palm is down
6. Supination: turning the forearm so the palm is up
7. Circumduction: moving the arm in a circle around the shoulder
8. Inversion: moving the sole of the foot inward at the ankle
9. Eversion: moving the sole of the foot outward at the ankle
10. Rotation: moving the head around a central axis
11. Protraction: moving a body part forward and parallel to the ground
12. Retraction: moving a body part backward and parallel to the ground
13. Elevation: raising a body part
14. Depression: lowering a body part

The **vertebrae** are 33 connecting bones stacked in a vertical column (Fig. 15.3). The vertebral column has four curves (a double-S shape). The cervical and lumbar curves are concave (inward or anterior), and the thoracic and sacrococcygeal curves are convex. The balanced or compensatory nature of these curves, together with the resilient intervertebral discs, allows the spine to absorb a great deal of shock.

SOCIAL DETERMINANTS OF HEALTH CONSIDERATIONS

Arthritis is one of the most prevalent chronic health conditions and a leading cause of pain, physical disability, and health care utilization in Canada;

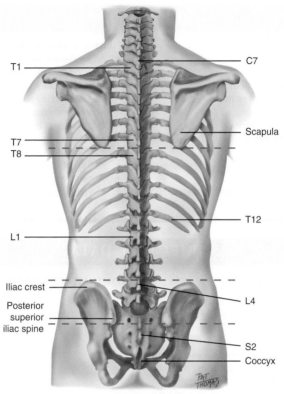

T1

C7

Scapula

T7
T8

T12

L1

Iliac crest

L4

Posterior
superior
iliac spine

S2

Coccyx

PAT
THOMAS

LANDMARKS OF THE SPINE

15.3

in 2016, about 6.1 million Canadians (20.4%) aged 15 and older reported that they had arthritis (Statistics Canada, 2017). In that year, arthritis was prevalent among 23.9% of females and 17.3% of males. The prevalence of arthritis increases with age, and the highest number of people affected are 75 years and older (Public Health Agency of Canada, 2011). For individuals who are under 65, this condition frequently results in loss of work and productivity. Prevalence of arthritis is higher among women; individuals living in rural areas; people with lower education

and income level; and is 1.3 to 1.6 times higher among First Nations and Métis adults.

Osteoarthritis is the most prevalent type of arthritis, affecting more than 3 million Canadians (Arthritis Society, 2015). Risk factors for osteoarthritis include increasing age, family history, excess weight, and joint injury. About 300,000 Canadians have rheumatoid arthritis; three times more women than men are affected (Arthritis Society, 2015). The cause of rheumatoid arthritis is unknown, and it can occur at any age, but it usually appears between the ages of 40 and 60.

SUBJECTIVE DATA

1. Joints
   - Pain
   - Stiffness
   - Swelling, heat, redness
   - Limitation of movement
2. Muscles
   - Pain (cramps)
   - Weakness
3. Bones
   - Pain
   - Deformity
   - Trauma (fractures, sprains, dislocations)
4. Functional assessment (ADLs)
   - Any self-care deficit in bathing, toileting, dressing, grooming, eating, mobility, communicating
   - Use of mobility aids
5. Self-care behaviours
   - Occupational hazards
     - Heavy lifting
     - Repetitive motion to joints
   - Nature of exercise program
   - Recent weight gain
   - Medications

OBJECTIVE DATA

PREPARATION

The purpose of the musculo-skeletal examination is to assess function for ADLs, as well as to screen for any abnormalities.

A screening musculo-skeletal examination suffices for most patients:
- Inspection and palpation of joints integrated with inspection of each body region
- Observation of range of motion (ROM) as patient proceeds through motions described earlier
- Age-specific screening measures (e.g., scoliosis screening for adolescents)

A **complete musculo-skeletal examination,** as described in this chapter, is appropriate for patients with articular disease, a history of musculo-skeletal symptoms, or any problems with ADLs.

EQUIPMENT NEEDED

Tape measure
Skin-marking pen

Normal Range of Findings	Abnormal Findings
Order of the Examination	
Inspection	
Compare corresponding paired joints. Inspect for symmetry of structure and function, as well as normal parameters for each joint.	

Normal Range of Findings	Abnormal Findings
Note the *size* and *contour* of the joint. Inspect the skin and tissues over the joints for *colour, swelling,* and *masses* or *deformity*.	Swelling may be caused by excess joint fluid (effusion), thickening of the synovial lining, inflammation of surrounding soft tissue (bursae, tendons), or bony enlargement.
	Deformities include **dislocation** (one or more bones in a joint being out of position), **subluxation** (partial dislocation of a joint), **contracture** (shortening of a muscle leading to limited ROM of joint), or **ankylosis** (stiffness or fixation of a joint).

Palpation

Palpate each joint, including its skin, for temperature, its muscles, bony articulations, and area of joint capsule. Note any heat, tenderness, swelling, and masses. Joints are normally not tender to palpation.

Warmth and tenderness signal inflammation.

Range of Motion

Ask for **active (voluntary) ROM** while stabilizing the body area proximal to that being moved. Familiarize yourself with the type of each joint and its normal ROM so you can recognize limitations.

If you see a limitation, gently attempt **passive motion:** anchor the joint with one hand while your other hand slowly moves it to its limit. The normal ranges of active and passive motion should be the same.

Joint motion normally causes no tenderness, pain, or crepitation. Do not confuse crepitation with the normal, discrete "crack" heard as a tendon or ligament slips over bone during motion, such as a knee bend.

Articular disease (inside the joint capsule, such as arthritis) produces swelling and tenderness around the whole joint, and limits both active and passive ROM in all planes. **Extra-articular** disease (injury to a specific tendon, ligament, nerve) produces swelling and tenderness to that one spot in the joint and affects ROM in only certain planes, especially during active (voluntary) motion.

Crepitation is an audible and palpable crunching or grating that accompanies movement. Crepitation occurs when the articular surfaces in the joints are roughened, as with rheumatoid arthritis.

Continued

Normal Range of Findings	Abnormal Findings

Muscle Testing

Test the strength of the prime mover muscle groups for each joint. Repeat the motions you elicited for active ROM. Ask the patient to flex (tighten or contract) the muscle and hold as you apply opposing force. Muscle strength should be equal bilaterally and should fully resist your opposing force. (Note: Muscle status and joint status are interdependent, and should be interpreted together. Chapter 16 discusses the examination of muscles for size, strength, tone, and involuntary movements.)

Strength varies widely among people. You may wish to use a grading system from "no voluntary movement" to "full strength," as shown in Table 15.1.

Cervical Spine

Inspect the alignment of head and neck. The spine should be straight and the head erect. *Palpate* the spinous processes and the sternomastoid, trapezius, and paravertebral muscles. They should feel firm, with no muscle spasm or tenderness.

Test ROM as follows*:

Head tilted to one side.
Asymmetry of muscles.
Tenderness and hard muscles with muscle spasm.

INSTRUCTIONS TO PATIENT	MOTION AND EXPECTED RANGE	
• Touch chin to chest.	Flexion of 45 degrees.	
• Lift the chin toward the ceiling.	Hyperextension of 55 degrees.	
• Move each ear toward the corresponding shoulder. Do not lift up the shoulder.	Lateral bending of 40 degrees.	
• Turn the chin toward each shoulder.	Rotation of 70 degrees.	

Limited ROM.
Pain with movement.

*Do not attempt if you suspect neck trauma.

Normal Range of Findings	Abnormal Findings
Ask the patient to repeat the motions while you apply opposing force. The patient normally can maintain flexion against your full resistance. This also tests integrity of cranial nerve XI (spinal nerve).	The patient cannot maintain flexion.

Upper Extremity

Shoulders

Inspect and compare both shoulders posteriorly and anteriorly. Check the size and contour of the joint and compare shoulders for equality of bony landmarks. There is normally no redness, muscular atrophy, deformity, or swelling present.	Redness. Inequality of bony landmarks. Atrophy manifesting as lack of fullness. Dislocated shoulder: loses the normal rounded shape and looks flattened laterally. Swelling from excess fluid: best seen anteriorly; considerable fluid must be present to cause a visible distension because the capsule is normally loose. (See Table 24.3, p. 674, in Jarvis: *Physical Examination and Health Assessment*, 3rd Canadian edition.)
While standing in front of the patient, *palpate* both shoulders, noting any muscular spasm or atrophy, swelling, heat, or tenderness.	Swelling. Hard muscles with muscle spasm. Tenderness or pain.
Test ROM by asking the patient to perform four motions. Cup one hand over the shoulder during ROM to note any crepitation; normally there is none.	

INSTRUCTIONS TO PATIENT	MOTION AND EXPECTED RANGE	
• With arms at sides and elbows extended, move both arms forward and up in wide vertical arcs. Then move them back.	Forward flexion of 180 degrees. Hyperextension up to 50 degrees.	Limited ROM. Asymmetry. Pain with motion. Crepitus with motion.

Continued

Normal Range of Findings	Abnormal Findings

INSTRUCTIONS TO PATIENT — **MOTION AND EXPECTED RANGE**

Instructions to Patient	Motion and Expected Range
• Rotate arms internally behind back, place back of hands as high as possible toward the scapulae.	Internal rotation of 90 degrees.
• With arms at sides and elbows extended, raise both arms in wide arcs in the coronal plane. Touch palms together above head.	Abduction of 180 degrees. Adduction of 50 degrees.
• Touch both hands behind the head, with elbows flexed and rotated posteriorly.	External rotation of 90 degrees.

Rotator cuff lesions may cause limited ROM, pain, and muscle spasm during abduction, whereas forward flexion stays fairly normal.

Test the strength of the shoulder muscles by asking the patient to shrug his or her shoulders, flex forward and up, and abduct against your resistance. The shoulder shrug also tests the integrity of cranial nerve XI (spinal nerve).

Elbow

Inspect the size and contour of the elbow in both flexed and extended positions. Look for any deformity, redness, or swelling.

Test ROM as follows:

Swelling and redness. (See Table 24.4, p. 675, in Jarvis: *Physical Examination and Health Assessment,* 3rd Canadian edition.)

Instructions to Patient	Motion and Expected Range
• Bend and straighten the elbow.	Flexion of 150 to 160 degrees, extension at 0. Some healthy people lack 5 to 10 degrees of full extension, and others have 5 to 10 degrees of hyperextension.
• Hold the hand midway; then touch front and back sides of hand to table.	Movement of 90 degrees in pronation and supination.

Normal Range of Findings	Abnormal Findings

While testing *muscle strength*, stabilize the patient's arm with one hand (Fig. 15.4). Have the patient flex the elbow against your resistance, applied just proximal to the wrist. Then ask the patient to extend the elbow against your resistance.

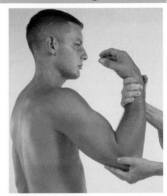

15.4 Stabilize the joint while testing muscle strength.

Wrist and Hand

Inspect the hands and wrists on the dorsal and palmar sides, noting position, contour, and shape. The normal functional position of the hand shows the wrist in slight extension. This way the fingers can flex efficiently, and the thumb can oppose them for grip and manipulation. The fingers lie straight in the same axis as the forearm. There is normally no swelling or redness, deformity, or nodules.

The skin looks smooth, with knuckle wrinkles present and no swelling or lesions. Muscles are full, with the palm showing a rounded mound proximal to the thumb (the *thenar eminence*), and a smaller rounded mound proximal to the little finger.

Palpate each joint in the wrist and hands. Facing the patient, support the hand with your fingers under it. Use gentle but firm pressure. Normally, the joint surfaces feel smooth, with no swelling, bogginess, nodules, or tenderness.

Subluxation of wrist.
Ulnar deviation: fingers list to ulnar side.
Ankylosis: wrist in extreme flexion.
Dupuytren's contracture: flexion contracture of one or more fingers.
Swan-neck or boutonnière deformity in fingers.
Atrophy of thenar eminence occurs with carpal tunnel syndrome as a result of compression of the median nerve.

Ganglion cyst in wrist.
Synovial swelling on dorsum.
Generalized swelling.
Tenderness.

Continued

Normal Range of Findings	Abnormal Findings

Test ROM as follows:

INSTRUCTIONS TO PATIENT	MOTION AND EXPECTED RANGE
• Bend the hand up at the wrist.	Hyperextension of 70 degrees.
• Bend hand down at the wrist.	Palmar flexion of 90 degrees.
• Bend the fingers up and down at metacarpophalangeal joints.	Flexion of 90 degrees. Hyperextension of 30 degrees.
• With palms flat on table, turn them outward and in.	Ulnar deviation of 50 to 60 degrees. Radial deviation of 20 degrees.
• Spread fingers apart; make a fist.	Abduction of 20 degrees; fist tight. The responses should be equal bilaterally.
• Touch the thumb to each finger and to the base of little finger.	The person is able to perform this manoeuvre, and the responses are equal bilaterally.

Loss of ROM here is the most common and the most significant type of function loss of the wrist.
Limited motion.
Pain on movement.

Lower Extremity

Hip

Inspect the hip joint together with the spine a bit later in the examination as the patient stands. At that time, note symmetrical levels of iliac crests, gluteal folds, and equal-sized buttocks. A smooth, even gait reflects equal leg lengths and functional hip motion.

Help the patient into a supine position, and *palpate* the hip joints. The joints should feel stable and symmetrical, with no tenderness or crepitation.

Pain with palpation.
Crepitation.

Test ROM as follows:

INSTRUCTIONS TO PATIENT	MOTION AND EXPECTED RANGE
• Raise each leg with knee extended.	Hip flexion of 90 degrees.

Limited motion.
Pain with motion.

Normal Range of Findings	Abnormal Findings

INSTRUCTIONS TO PATIENT	MOTION AND EXPECTED RANGE	
• Bend each knee up to the chest while keeping the other leg straight.	Hip flexion of 120 degrees. The opposite thigh should remain on the table.	Flexion flattens the lumbar spine; if this reveals a flexion deformity in the opposite hip, it represents a positive sign of the *Thomas test.*
• Flex knee and hip to 90 degrees. Stabilize by holding the thigh with one hand and the ankle with the other hand. Swing the foot outward. Swing the foot inward. (Foot and thigh move in opposing directions.)	Internal rotation of 40 degrees. External rotation of 45 degrees.	Limited internal rotation of hip is an early and reliable sign of hip disease.
• Swing leg laterally, then medially, with knee straight. Stabilize pelvis by pushing down on the opposite anterior superior iliac spine.	Abduction of 40 to 45 degrees. Adduction of 20 to 30 degrees.	Limitation of abduction of the hip, while supine, is the most common motion dysfunction found in hip disease.
• When standing (later in examination), swing straight leg back behind body. Stabilize pelvis to eliminate exaggerated lumbar lordosis.	Hyperextension of 15 degrees when stabilized.	

Knee

The skin normally looks smooth, with even colouring and no lesions.

Inspect lower leg alignment. The lower leg should extend in the same axis as the thigh.

Shiny and atrophic skin.
Swelling and inflammation.
Lesions (e.g., psoriasis).
Angulation deformity:
• Flexion contracture
• Genu valgum (knock knees)
• Genu varum (bow legs)

Continued

Normal Range of Findings	Abnormal Findings
Inspect the knee's shape and contour. Normally there are distinct concavities, or hollows, on either side of the patella. Check them for any sign of fullness or swelling. Check other locations, such as the prepatellar bursa and the suprapatellar pouch, for any abnormal swelling.	With synovial thickening or effusion, hollows disappear; then they may bulge. (See Table 24.6, p. 679, in Jarvis: *Physical Examination and Health Assessment*, 3rd Canadian edition.)
Check for any atrophy in the quadriceps muscle in the anterior thigh. Because it is the prime mover of knee extension, this muscle is important for joint stability during weight-bearing.	Atrophy occurs with disuse or chronic disorders. It first appears in the medial part of the muscle, although it is difficult to note because the vastus medialis is relatively small.

Test ROM as follows:

INSTRUCTIONS TO PATIENT	MOTION AND EXPECTED RANGE	
• Bend each knee.	Flexion of 130 to 150 degrees.	Limited ROM. Contracture. Pain with motion. Limpness.
• Extend each knee.	A straight line of 0 degrees, in some patients; a hyperextension of 15 degrees in others.	
• Check knee ROM during ambulation.		

Check muscle strength by asking the patient to maintain knee flexion while you oppose by trying to pull the leg forward. Muscle extension is demonstrated by the patient's success in rising from a seated position in a low chair or by rising from a squat without using the hands for support.	Sudden locking: the patient is unable to extend the knee fully. This usually occurs with a painful and audible "pop" or "click." Sudden buckling, or "giving way," occurs with ligament injury, which causes weakness and instability.

Normal Range of Findings	Abnormal Findings

Ankle and Foot

Inspect and compare both feet, noting position of feet and toes, contour of joints, and skin characteristics. The foot should align with the long axis of the lower leg.

Weight bearing should be borne on the middle of the foot, from the heel, along the midfoot, to between the second and third toes.

The toes point straight forward and lie flat. The ankles (malleoli) are smooth, bony prominences. The skin is normally smooth, with even colouring and no lesions. Note the locations of any calluses or bursal reactions because they reveal areas of abnormal friction. Examining well-worn shoes helps assess areas of wear and accommodation.

Test ROM as follows:

INSTRUCTIONS TO PATIENT	MOTION AND EXPECTED RANGE
• Point toes toward the floor.	Plantar flexion of 45 degrees.
• Point toes toward your nose.	Dorsiflexion of 20 degrees.
• Turn soles of feet out, then in. (Examiner stabilizes the ankle with one hand, hold heel with the other to test the subtalar joint.)	Eversion of 20 degrees. Inversion of 30 degrees.
• Flex and straighten toes.	

Assess muscle strength by asking the patient to maintain dorsiflexion and plantar flexion against your resistance.

Abnormal Findings column:

Hallux valgus (distal part of the great toe is directed *away* from the body midline).

Hammer toes; claw toes.

Swelling or inflammation.

Calluses; ulcers.

(See Table 24.7, p. 682, in Jarvis: *Physical Examination and Health Assessment,* 3rd Canadian edition.)

Limited ROM.
Pain with motion.

The patient cannot maintain flexion.

Continued

Normal Range of Findings	Abnormal Findings

Spine

The patient should be standing, draped in a gown open at the back. Place yourself far enough back so that you can see the entire back. *Inspect* and note if the spine is straight by following an imaginary vertical line from the head through the spinous processes and down through the gluteal cleft; by noting equal horizontal positions for the shoulders, scapulae, iliac crests, and gluteal folds; and by noting equal spaces between the arm and lateral thorax on the two sides (Fig. 15.5, *A*). The patient's knees and feet should be aligned with the trunk and should be pointing forward.

A difference in shoulder elevation and in level of scapulae and iliac crests occurs with scoliosis (Table 15.2).

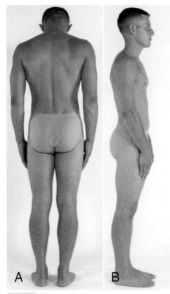

15.5 **A.** Straight spine. **B.** Normal curvature seen from side.

Normal Range of Findings	Abnormal Findings
From the side, note the normal convex thoracic curve and concave lumbar curve (Fig. 15.5, *B*). An enhanced thoracic curve, or **kyphosis,** is common in older adults. A pronounced lumbar curve, or **lordosis,** is common in obese people.	Lateral tilting and forward bending occur with a herniated nucleus pulposus (see Table 15.2).

Test ROM of the spine by asking the patient to bend forward and touch the toes. Look for flexion of 75 to 90 degrees and smoothness and symmetry of movement. Note that the concave lumbar curve should disappear with this motion, and the back should have a single, convex, C-shaped curve.

Stabilize the pelvis with your hands. *Test ROM* as follows:

INSTRUCTIONS TO PATIENT	MOTION AND EXPECTED RANGE
Bend sideways.	Lateral bending of 35 degrees.
Bend backward.	Hyperextension of 30 degrees.
Twist shoulders to one side, then the other.	Rotation of 30 degrees, bilaterally.

Limited ROM.

Pain with motion.

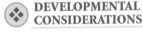

❖ DEVELOPMENTAL CONSIDERATIONS

Infants

Lift up the infant and examine the back. Note the normal, single, C-curve of the newborn's spine (Fig. 15.6). By 2 months of age, the infant can lift the head while prone. This builds the concave cervical spinal curve and indicates normal forearm strength.

Observe ROM through spontaneous movement of extremities.

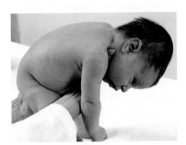

15.6 Normal spinal curvature in newborn.

Continued

Normal Range of Findings	Abnormal Findings
Test muscle strength by lifting up the infant with your hands under the baby's axillae. A baby with normal muscle strength wedges securely between your hands.	A baby who starts to "slip" between your hands shows weakness of the shoulder muscles.

Preschool-Age and School-Age Children

Once the infant learns to crawl and then to walk, the waking hours are spent seemingly in perpetual motion. This is convenient for your musculo-skeletal assessment; you can observe the muscles and joints during spontaneous play before a table-top examination. Most young children enjoy showing off their physical accomplishments. For specific motions, coax the toddler: "Show me how you can walk to Mom," or "Climb the stepstool." Ask the preschooler to hop on one foot or to jump.

While the child is standing, note the posture. From behind, you should note a "plumb line" from the back of the head, along the spine, to the middle of the sacrum. Shoulders are level within 1 cm and scapulae are symmetrical. From the side, lordosis is common throughout childhood, appearing more pronounced in children with a protuberant abdomen.

Check the child's gait while the child walks away from and toward you. Let the child wear socks, because a cold tile floor will distort the usual gait.

From 1 to 2 years of age, expect a broad-based gait, with arms out for balance. Weight bearing is borne on the inside of the foot. From 3 years of age, the base narrows and the arms are closer to the sides. Inspect the shoes for spots of greatest wear to aid your judgement of the gait. Normally, the shoes wear more on the outside of the heel and the inside of the toe.

Abnormal column findings:

Lordosis is marked with muscular dystrophy and rickets.

Limp; usually caused by trauma, fatigue, or hip disease.

Abnormal gait patterns.

Normal Range of Findings	Abnormal Findings

Adolescents

Proceed with the musculo-skeletal examination as for the adult, except pay special note to spinal posture. Kyphosis is common during adolescence because of chronic poor posture. Be aware of the risk of sports-related injuries with the adolescent because sports participation and competition reach a height with this age group.

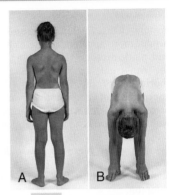

15.7 Scoliosis screening.

Inspect for scoliosis with the *forward bend test* (Fig. 15.7). Seat yourself behind the standing child, and ask the child stand with feet shoulder-width apart and to bend forward to touch the toes. Expect a straight vertical spine while standing and also while bending forward. Posterior ribs should be symmetrical, with equal elevation of shoulders, scapulae, and iliac crests. You may wish to mark each spinous process with a felt marker when the adolescent bends forward. The lineup of ink dots when she or he stands up highlights even a subtle curve.

Scoliosis is most apparent during the preadolescent growth spurt. Asymmetry is suggestive of scoliosis: the ribs "hump up" on one side as child bends forward and landmark elevation is unequal (see Table 15.2).

Pregnant Women

Proceed through the examination described for adults. Expected postural changes in pregnancy include progressive lordosis and, toward the third trimester, anterior cervical flexion, kyphosis, and slumped shoulders (Fig. 15.8, *A*). At full term, the protuberant abdomen and the relaxed mobility in the joints create the characteristic waddling gait (Fig. 15.8, *B*).

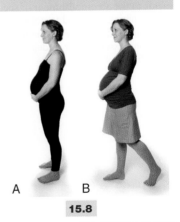

A   B

15.8

Continued

Normal Range of Findings	Abnormal Findings

Older Adults

Postural changes include a decrease in height, more apparent in the eighth and ninth decades. "Lengthening of the arm–trunk axis" describes this shortening of the trunk with the appearance of comparatively long extremities. Kyphosis is common, with a backward head tilt to compensate. This creates the outline of a figure 3 when you view this older adult from the left side (Fig. 15.9). Slight flexion of hips and knees is also common.

Contour changes include a decrease of fat in the body periphery and fat deposition over the abdomen and hips. The bony prominences become more marked.

ROM and muscle strength are much the same as with younger adults provided there are no musculo-skeletal illnesses or arthritic changes.

Functional Assessment

For those with advanced aging changes, arthritic changes, or musculo-skeletal disability, perform a functional assessment for ADLs. This applies the ROM and muscle strength assessments to the accomplishment of specific activities. You need to determine adequate and safe performance of functions essential for independent home life.

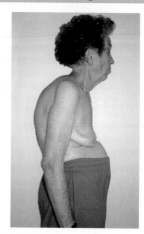

15.9 Postural changes with aging.

INSTRUCTIONS TO PATIENT	COMMON ADAPTATION TO AGING CHANGES	INSTRUCTIONS TO PATIENT	COMMON ADAPTATION TO AGING CHANGES
• Walk (with shoes on).	Shuffling pattern; swaying; arms out to help balance; broader base of support; watching own feet.	• Pick up object from floor.	Person often bends at waist instead of at the knees; holds furniture for support while bending and straightening.
• Climb up stairs.	Person holds hand rail; may haul body up with arm; may lead with favoured (stronger) leg.	• Rise up from sitting in a chair.	Person uses arms to push off chair arms, upper trunk leans forward before body straightens, feet planted wide in broad base of support.
• Walk down stairs.	Holds hand rail tightly, sometimes with both hands. If the person is weak, he or she may descend sideways, lowering the weaker leg first. If the person is unsteady, he or she may watch feet.	• Rise up from lying in bed.	May roll to one side, push with arms to lift up torso, grab bedside table to increase leverage.

Summary Checklist: Musculo-Skeletal System Examination

For each joint to be examined:
1. **Inspection:**
   Size and contour of joint
   Skin colour and characteristics
2. **Palpation of joint area:**
   Skin
   Muscles

Bony articulations
Joint capsule
3. **ROM:**
   Active
   Passive (if active ROM is limited)
4. **Muscle testing**
5. **Engage in teaching and health promotion**

ABNORMAL FINDINGS

TABLE 15.1	Grading Muscle Strength		
Grade	Description	Percent Normal	Assessment
5	Full ROM against gravity, full resistance	100	Normal
4	Full ROM against gravity, some resistance	75	Good
3	Full ROM with gravity	50	Fair
2	Full ROM with gravity eliminated (passive motion)	25	Poor
1	Slight contraction	10	Trace
0	No contraction	0	Zero

TABLE 15.2   Abnormalities of the Spine

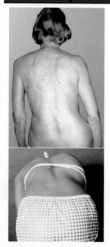

Scoliosis

Lateral curvature of thoracic and lumbar segments of the spine, usually with some rotation of involved vertebral bodies.

Functional scoliosis is flexible; it is apparent on standing and disappears on forward bending. It may be compensatory for other abnormalities such as leg length discrepancy.

Structural scoliosis is fixed; the curvature shows both on standing and on bending forward. In illustration, note rib hump with forward flexion. When the patient is standing, note unequal shoulder elevation, unequal scapulae, obvious curvature, and unequal hip level. At greatest risk are girls aged 10 years through adolescence, during the peak of the growth spurt.

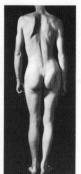

Herniated Nucleus Pulposus

The nucleus pulposus (at the centre of the intervertebral disc) ruptures into the spinal canal and puts pressure on the local spinal nerve root. It is usually caused by stress, such as lifting, twisting, continuous flexion with lifting, or a fall onto the buttocks. It occurs mostly in men 20–45 years of age. Lumbar herniations occur mainly in interspaces L4–L5 and L5–S1. Note sciatic pain, numbness, and paraesthesia of involved dermatome; listing away from affected side; decreased mobility; low back tenderness; and decreased motor and sensory function in leg. Straight leg raising tests reproduce sciatic pain.

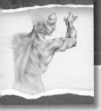

CHAPTER 16

Neurological System

STRUCTURE AND FUNCTION

The nervous system can be divided into two parts: central and peripheral. The **central nervous system (CNS)** includes the brain and spinal cord. The **peripheral nervous system** includes the 12 pairs of cranial nerves, the 31 pairs of spinal nerves, and all their branches. The peripheral nervous system carries sensory (afferent) messages *to* the CNS from sensory receptors and motor (efferent) messages *from* the CNS out to muscles and glands, as well as autonomic messages that govern the internal organs and blood vessels.

THE CENTRAL NERVOUS SYSTEM

The **cerebral cortex** is the cerebrum's outer layer of nerve cell bodies, also called "grey matter." The cerebral cortex (cerebrum) is the centre for humans' highest functions, governing thought, memory, reasoning, sensation, and voluntary movement (Fig. 16.1).

Each half of the cerebrum is a **hemisphere.** Each hemisphere is divided into four **lobes:** frontal, parietal, temporal, and occipital.

The lobes have certain areas that mediate specific functions as labelled in Figure 16.1. Damage to any of

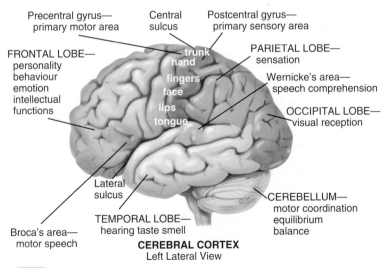

Precentral gyrus—
primary motor area

Central
sulcus

Postcentral gyrus—
primary sensory area

FRONTAL LOBE—
personality
behaviour
emotion
intellectual
functions

trunk
hand
fingers
face
lips
tongue

PARIETAL LOBE—
sensation

Wernicke's area—
speech comprehension

OCCIPITAL LOBE—
visual reception

Lateral
sulcus

Broca's area—
motor speech

TEMPORAL LOBE—
hearing taste smell

CEREBELLUM—
motor coordination
equilibrium
balance

CEREBRAL CORTEX
Left Lateral View

16.1 The lobes of the cerebral cortex and their specific functions. *(© Pat Thomas, 2006.)*

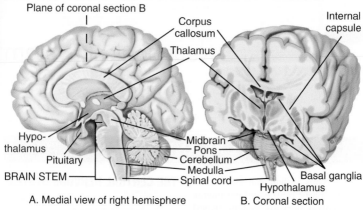

Plane of coronal section B

Corpus callosum

Internal capsule

Thalamus

Hypo-thalamus

Pituitary

BRAIN STEM

Midbrain
Pons
Cerebellum
Medulla
Spinal cord

Basal ganglia
Hypothalamus

A. Medial view of right hemisphere

B. Coronal section

COMPONENTS OF THE CENTRAL NERVOUS SYSTEM

16.2   *(© Pat Thomas, 2006.)*

these specific cortical areas produces a corresponding loss of function: motor weakness, paralysis, loss of sensation, or impaired ability to understand and process language.

In addition to the cerebral cortex, the CNS has other vital components (Fig. 16.2).

The **thalamus** is the main relay station for incoming sensory pathways.

The **hypothalamus** controls temperature, heart rate, and blood pressure; regulates sleep and the pituitary gland; and coordinates autonomic nervous system activity, and emotional status.

The **cerebellum** is concerned with motor coordination of voluntary movements, equilibrium, and muscle tone.

The **midbrain** and **pons** contain motor neurons, and motor and sensory tracts. The **medulla** contains fibre tracts and vital autonomic centres for respiratory, cardiac, and gastro-intestinal functions.

The **spinal cord** is the main pathway for ascending and descending fibre tracts that connect the brain to the spinal nerves, and it mediates reflexes.

THE PERIPHERAL NERVOUS SYSTEM

Reflex Arc

Reflexes are basic defence mechanisms of the nervous system. In the simplest reflex, the sensory afferent fibres carry the message from the receptor and travel through the dorsal root into the spinal cord (Fig. 16.3). They synapse directly in the cord with the motor neuron in the anterior horn. Motor efferent fibres leave via the ventral root and travel to the muscle, stimulating a sudden contraction.

The deep tendon (myotatic or stretch) reflex has five components:

1. An intact sensory nerve (afferent)
2. A functional synapse in the cord
3. An intact motor nerve fibre (efferent)
4. The neuromuscular junction
5. A competent muscle

Cranial Nerves

Cranial nerves enter and exit the brain rather than the spinal cord (Fig. 16.4). The 12 pairs of cranial nerves supply primarily the head and neck, with the

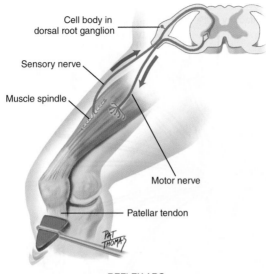

Cell body in
dorsal root ganglion

Sensory nerve

Muscle spindle

Motor nerve

Patellar tendon

REFLEX ARC

16.3 *(© Pat Thomas, 2006.)*

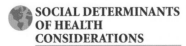

exception of the vagus nerve, which travels to the heart, respiratory muscles, stomach, and gallbladder.

Spinal Nerves

The 31 pairs of **spinal nerves** arise from the length of the spinal cord and supply the rest of the body (Fig. 16.5). They are named for the region of the spine from which they exit: 8 cervical, 12 thoracic, 5 lumbar, 5 sacral, and 1 coccygeal. They are "mixed" nerves because they contain both sensory and motor fibres.

A **dermatome** is a circumscribed skin area that is supplied mainly from one spinal cord segment through a particular spinal nerve.

🌐 SOCIAL DETERMINANTS OF HEALTH CONSIDERATIONS

As with all aspects of health, social determinants have an impact on

neurological health and related systems. Stroke is the third leading cause of death and the leading cause of disability in Canada. Each year, over 62 000 new cases of stroke occur in Canada (Blacquiere et al., 2017), with nearly 14 000 Canadians dying each year (Ontario Stroke Network, 2016). The prevalence of stroke increases with age and other risk factors, such as hypertension, smoking, and associated cardiac conditions, such as atrial fibrillation.

A stroke, or cerebrovascular accident, occurs when the blood flow is interrupted to a part of the brain, which is why it is often referred to as a "brain attack." The most common type is an *ischemic* stroke, in which a blood clot blocks a blood vessel in the brain. Less common is a *hemorrhagic* stroke, which occurs when a blood vessel in the brain ruptures and causes bleeding. The symptoms and after effects of a stroke depend on which area of the brain is affected and

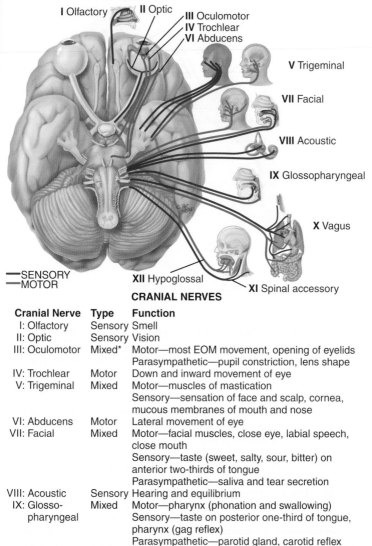

I Olfactory
II Optic
III Oculomotor
IV Trochlear
VI Abducens
V Trigeminal
VII Facial
VIII Acoustic
IX Glossopharyngeal
X Vagus
XII Hypoglossal
XI Spinal accessory

SENSORY
MOTOR

CRANIAL NERVES

Cranial Nerve	Type	Function
I: Olfactory	Sensory	Smell
II: Optic	Sensory	Vision
III: Oculomotor	Mixed*	Motor—most EOM movement, opening of eyelids Parasympathetic—pupil constriction, lens shape
IV: Trochlear	Motor	Down and inward movement of eye
V: Trigeminal	Mixed	Motor—muscles of mastication Sensory—sensation of face and scalp, cornea, mucous membranes of mouth and nose
VI: Abducens	Motor	Lateral movement of eye
VII: Facial	Mixed	Motor—facial muscles, close eye, labial speech, close mouth Sensory—taste (sweet, salty, sour, bitter) on anterior two-thirds of tongue Parasympathetic—saliva and tear secretion
VIII: Acoustic	Sensory	Hearing and equilibrium
IX: Glosso-pharyngeal	Mixed	Motor—pharynx (phonation and swallowing) Sensory—taste on posterior one-third of tongue, pharynx (gag reflex) Parasympathetic—parotid gland, carotid reflex
X: Vagus	Mixed	Motor—pharynx and larynx (talking and swallowing) Sensory—general sensation from carotid body, carotid sinus, pharynx, viscera Parasympathetic—carotid reflex
XI: Spinal	Motor	Movement of trapezius and sternomastoid muscles
XII: Hypoglossal	Motor	Movement of tongue

Mixed refers to a nerve carrying a combination of fibres: motor + sensory; motor + parasympathetic; or motor + sensory + parasympathetic.

16.4 *(© Pat Thomas, 2006.)*

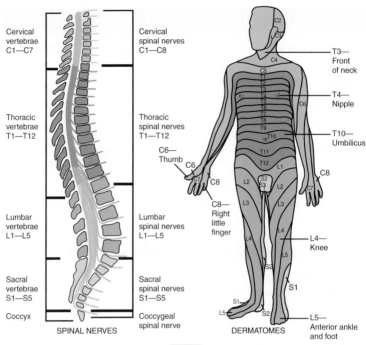

Cervical vertebrae C1—C7

Cervical spinal nerves C1—C8

Thoracic vertebrae T1—T12

Thoracic spinal nerves T1—T12

C6— Thumb

Lumbar vertebrae L1—L5

Lumbar spinal nerves L1—L5

C8— Right little finger

Sacral vertebrae S1—S5

Sacral spinal nerves S1—S5

Coccyx

Coccygeal spinal nerve

SPINAL NERVES

T3— Front of neck

T4— Nipple

T10— Umbilicus

L4— Knee

L5— Anterior ankle and foot

DERMATOMES

16.5

to what extent. This can make a stroke difficult to diagnose. However, early recognition of symptoms and prompt treatment are essential so that appropriate treatments and interventions can be initiated as soon as possible.

For more information about stroke and stroke prevention, see Chapter 25, page 695, in Jarvis: *Physical Examination and Health Assessment,* 3rd Canadian edition.

SUBJECTIVE DATA

1. Headache (unusually frequent or severe)
2. Head injury
3. Dizziness (feeling lightheaded or faint)/vertigo (feeling a rotational spinning)
4. Seizures
5. Tremors
6. Weakness
7. Incoordination

8. Numbness or tingling sensation
9. Difficulty swallowing
10. Difficulty speaking
11. Significant past history (stroke [brain attack], spinal cord injury, meningitis or encephalitis, congenital defect, alcoholism)
12. Environmental and occupational hazards

OBJECTIVE DATA

PREPARATION

Perform a **screening neurological examination** (items identified in following sections) of seemingly healthy patients whose histories reveal no significant subjective findings.

Perform a **neurological recheck examination** of patients with demonstrated neurological deficits who require periodic assessments (e.g., hospitalized patients or those in extended care), using the examination sequence beginning on page 12.

EQUIPMENT NEEDED

Penlight
Tongue blade
Cotton swab
Cotton ball
Tuning fork (128 or 256 Hz)
Percussion hammer
(Possibly) Familiar aromatic substances, such as peppermint, coffee, vanilla

Normal Range of Findings	Abnormal Findings
Mental Status	
Assess level of consciousness (see Chapter 2 and examination sequence on p. 12).	
Test Selected Cranial Nerves	
Cranial Nerve II: Optic Nerve	
Test visual acuity and test visual fields by confrontation. Use the ophthalmoscope to examine the ocular fundus to determine the colour, size, and shape of the optic disc (see Chapter 7).	Visual field loss. (See Table 15.5, p. 342, in Jarvis: *Physical Examination and Health Assessment,* 3rd Canadian edition.)
	Papilledema with increased intracranial pressure; optic atrophy. (See Table 15.9, p. 346, in Jarvis: *Physical Examination and Health Assessment,* 3rd Canadian edition.)
Cranial Nerves III, IV, and VI: Oculomotor, Trochlear, and Abducens Nerves	
Palpebral fissures are usually equal in width or nearly so.	Ptosis (drooping) with myasthenia gravis, dysfunction of cranial nerve III, or Horner's syndrome (see Table 7.2, p. 78).

Normal Range of Findings	Abnormal Findings
Check pupils for size, regularity, equality, direct and consensual light reactions, and accommodation (see Chapter 7). The pupils are normally equal, round, react to light promptly, and react to accommodation (PERRLA).	Unequal size, constricted pupils, dilated pupils, or no response to light (see Table 7.3, p. 80). Increasing intracranial pressure causes sudden, unilateral dilation and nonreactivity of a pupil.
Assess extraocular movements by the cardinal positions of gaze (see Chapter 7).	Strabismus (deviated gaze) or limited movement.
Nystagmus is a back-and-forth oscillation of the eyes. End-point nystagmus, a few beats of horizontal nystagmus at extreme lateral gaze, is normal. Assess any other nystagmus carefully.	Nystagmus occurs with disease of the vestibular system, cerebellum, or brain stem.

Cranial Nerve V: Trigeminal Nerve

Motor Function. Palpate the temporal and masseter muscles as the patient clenches the teeth. Muscles should feel equally strong on both sides. Try to separate the jaws by pushing down on the chin; normally you cannot.

Decreased strength on one or both sides.
Asymmetry in jaw movement.
Pain with clenching of teeth.

Sensory Function. With the patient's eyes closed, test light touch sensation by touching a cotton wisp on designated areas of the patient's face: forehead, cheeks, and chin. Ask the patient to say "now" whenever the touch is felt.

Decreased or unequal sensation.

Cranial Nerve VII: Facial Nerve

Motor Function. Note mobility and facial symmetry as the patient responds to these requests: smile, frown, close eyes tightly (against your attempt to open them), lift eyebrows, show teeth, and puff cheeks.

Muscle weakness is demonstrated by loss of the nasolabial fold, drooping of one side of the face, lower eyelid sagging, and escape of air from only one puffed cheek when both are pressed in. Loss of movement and asymmetry of movement occur both with CNS lesions (e.g., cerebrovascular accident that affects the lower face on one side) and with lesions of the peripheral nervous system (e.g., cases of Bell's palsy that affect the upper *and* lower portions of one side of the face).

Continued

Normal Range of Findings	Abnormal Findings

Cranial Nerve VIII: Acoustic (Vestibulocochlear) Nerve

Test hearing acuity by patient's ability to hear normal conversation and by the whispered voice test (see Chapter 8).

Cranial Nerves IX and X: Glossopharyngeal and Vagus Nerves

Motor Function. Depress the tongue with a tongue blade and note movement as the patient says "ahh" or yawns; uvula and soft palate should rise in the midline, and tonsillar pillars move medially.

Absence or asymmetry of soft palate movement.
Deviation of uvula to side.
Asymmetry of tonsillar pillar movement.

Cranial Nerve XI: Spinal Accessory Nerve

Check strength of neck muscles by asking patient to rotate head forcibly against your resistance at side of chin and to shrug shoulders against resistance. Both sides should feel equally strong.

Atrophy.
Muscle weakness or paralysis.

Cranial Nerve XII: Hypoglossal Nerve

Note the forward thrust in the midline as the patient sticks out the tongue. Ask patient to say, "light, tight, dynamite"; lingual speech (sounds of letters *l, t, d, n*) should be clear and distinct.

Atrophy: fasciculations (see Table 16.1).
Tongue deviates to side with lesions of the hypoglossal nerve. (When this occurs, deviation is toward the paralyzed side.)

Inspect and Palpate the Motor System

Muscles

Size. Muscle groups should be within the normal size limits for age and should be symmetrical bilaterally. When muscles in the extremities look asymmetrical, measure each in centimetres, and record the difference. A difference of 1 cm or less is not significant. Note that it is difficult to assess muscle mass in very obese patients.

Atrophy: abnormally small muscle with a wasted appearance; occurs with disuse, injury, lower motor neuron disease, such as polio, diabetic neuropathy.
Hypertrophy: increased size and strength; occurs with isometric exercise.

Normal Range of Findings	Abnormal Findings
Strength. Test homologous muscles simultaneously (see Chapter 15). Test muscle groups of the extremities, neck, and trunk.	Paresis (weakness) is diminished strength; paralysis (plegia) is absence of strength (see Table 16.1).

Cerebellar Function

Normal Range of Findings	Abnormal Findings
Gait. Observe as the patient walks 3 to 6 m, turns, and returns to the starting point. Normally, the gait is smooth, rhythmic, and effortless; the opposing arm swing is coordinated; turns are smooth. The step length is about 30 cm from heel to heel. Ask the patient to walk a straight line in a heel-to-toe manner (tandem walking) (Fig. 16.6). This decreases the base of support and accentuates any problem with coordination. Normally, patient person can walk straight and stay balanced.	Stiff, immobile posture; staggering or reeling; wide base of support. Lack of arm swing or rigid arms. Unequal rhythm of steps; slapping of foot; scraping of toe of shoe. Ataxia: uncoordinated or unsteady gait. Crooked line of walk. Widens base to maintain balance. Staggering, reeling, or loss of balance. An ataxia that did not appear with regular gait may now appear. Inability to tandem walk is indicative of an upper motor neuron lesion, such as multiple sclerosis, or acute cerebellar dysfunction, as with alcohol intoxication.
Romberg Test. Ask the patient to stand with feet together and arms at the sides. Once in a stable position, ask the patient to close the eyes and hold the position (Fig. 16.7). Wait about 20 seconds. Normally, a patient can maintain posture and balance even with the visual orienting information blocked, although there may be slight swaying. (Stand close to catch the patient in case he or she falls.)	Swaying, falling, widening base of feet to avoid falling. *Positive* Romberg sign is loss of balance that occurs when the eyes are closed. It occurs with cerebellar ataxia (multiple sclerosis, alcohol intoxication), loss of proprioception, and loss of vestibular function.
Ask the patient to perform a shallow knee bend or to hop in place, first on one leg, then the other. This demonstrates normal position sense, muscle strength, and cerebellar function. Note that some individuals cannot hop because of aging or obesity.	Inability to perform knee bend because of weakness in quadriceps muscle or hip extensors.

Continued

Normal Range of Findings	Abnormal Findings

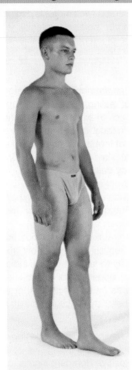

16.6 Tandem walking.

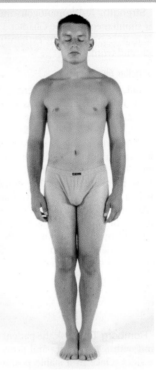

16.7 Romberg test.

Assess the Sensory System

Make sure the patient is alert, cooperative, and comfortable, and has an adequate attention span; otherwise, you may get misleading and invalid results. Testing of the sensory system can be fatiguing. You may need to repeat the examination later or conduct only parts of it when the patient is tired.

Routine screening procedures include testing superficial pain, light touch, vibration in a few distal locations, and testing stereognosis.

The patient's eyes should be closed during each test. Take time to explain what will be happening and exactly how you expect the patient to respond.

Normal Range of Findings	Abnormal Findings

Pain

Break a tongue blade lengthwise, forming a sharp point at the fractured end and a dull spot at the rounded end. Lightly apply the sharp point or the dull end to the patient's body in a random, unpredictable order (Fig. 16.8A and B). Ask the patient to say "sharp" or "dull," depending on the sensation felt. (Note that the sharp edge is used to test for pain; the dull edge is used as a general test of the patient's responses.)

Let at least 2 seconds elapse between each stimulus to avoid *summation*. With summation, frequent consecutive stimuli are perceived as one strong stimulus.

Hypoalgesia: decreased pain sensation.

Analgesia: absent pain sensation.

Hyperalgesia: increased pain sensation.

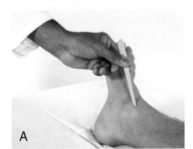 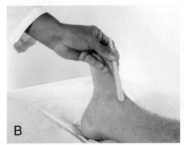

16.8 Test superficial pain.

Light Touch

Apply a wisp of cotton to the skin. Stretch a cotton ball to lengthen it, and brush it over the skin in a random order of sites and at irregular intervals. Ask the patient to say "now" or "yes" when touch is felt. Compare symmetrical points.

Hypoesthesia: decreased touch sensation.

Anaesthesia: absent touch sensation.

Hyperesthesia: increased touch sensation.

Continued

Normal Range of Findings	Abnormal Findings

Vibration

Strike a low-pitched tuning fork on the heel of your hand and hold the base on a bony surface of the patient's fingers and great toe. Ask the patient to indicate when the vibration starts and stops. The normal response is vibration or a buzzing sensation on these distal areas. If no vibrations are felt, move proximally and test ulnar processes, ankles, patellae, and iliac crests. Compare responses on the right side to the left. If you find a deficit, note whether it is gradual or abrupt.

Inability to feel vibration: loss of vibration sense occurs with peripheral neuropathy, for example, diabetes and alcoholism. This is often the first sensation lost.

Peripheral neuropathy is worst at the feet, and sensation gradually improves up the leg, whereas a specific nerve lesion produces a clear zone of deficit for its dermatome.

Tactile Discrimination (Fine Touch)

Stereognosis. Test the patient's ability to recognize objects by feeling their forms, sizes, and weights, with eyes closed. Place a familiar object (paper clip, key, coin, cotton ball, or pencil) in the patient's hand and ask the patient to identify it (Fig. 16.9). A patient will normally explore it with the fingers and correctly name it. Test a different object in each hand; testing the left hand helps you assess functioning of the right parietal lobe.

Problems with tactile discrimination occur with lesions of the sensory cortex or posterior column.

Astereognosis (inability to identify object correctly) occurs with sensory cortex lesions, such as cerebrovascular attack (stroke).

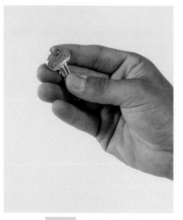

16.9 Stereognosis.

Normal Range of Findings	Abnormal Findings

Test the Reflexes

Stretch (Deep Tendon) Reflexes

For an adequate response, the limb should be relaxed and the muscle partially stretched. Stimulate the reflex by directing a short, snappy blow of the reflex hammer onto the muscle's insertion tendon. Strike a brief, well-aimed blow and bounce up promptly; do not let the hammer rest on the tendon. Use the pointed end of the reflex hammer when aiming at a smaller target (such as your thumb) on the tendon site; use the flat end when the target is wider or to diffuse the impact and prevent pain.

Use just enough force to get a response. Compare right and left sides; the responses should be equal. The reflex response is graded on a five-point scale:

4+ : Very brisk, hyperactive with clonus; indicative of disease
3+ : Brisker than average; may indicate disease
2+ : Average; normal
1+ : Diminished; low normal
0 : No response

Clonus is a set of rapid, rhythmic contractions of the same muscle.

Hyperreflexia is the exaggerated reflex that occurs when the monosynaptic reflex arc is released from the usually inhibiting influence of higher cortical levels. This occurs with upper motor neuron lesions, such as a cerebrovascular accident.

Hyporeflexia, the reduced functioning of a reflex, is a lower motor neuron problem. In some cases, the reflex may be absent. It results from interruption of sensory afferent pathways or destruction of motor efferent fibres and anterior horn cells, as in spinal cord injury.

Biceps Reflex (C5 to C6). Support the patient's forearm on yours; this position relaxes and partially flexes the patient's arm. Place your thumb on the biceps tendon and strike a blow on your thumb. You can feel as well as see the normal response, which is contraction of the biceps muscle and flexion of the forearm (Fig. 16.10).

Continued

Normal Range of Findings	Abnormal Findings

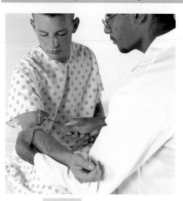

16.10 Biceps reflex.

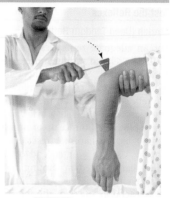

16.11 Triceps reflex.

Triceps Reflex (C7 to C8). Tell the patient to let the arm "just go limp" as you suspend it by holding the upper arm. Strike the triceps tendon directly just above the elbow (Fig. 16.11). The normal response is extension of the forearm. Alternatively, hold the patient's wrist across the chest to flex the arm at the elbow, and tap the tendon.

Quadriceps or Patellar ("Knee Jerk") Reflex (L2 to L4). Let the lower legs dangle freely to flex the knee and stretch the tendons. Strike the tendon directly just below the patella (Fig. 16.12). Extension of the lower leg is the expected response. Contraction of the quadriceps will also be palpable.

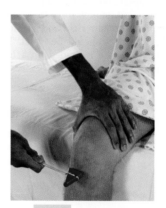

16.12 Patellar reflex.

Achilles ("Ankle Jerk") Reflex (L5 to S2). Position the patient with the knee flexed and the hip externally rotated. Hold the foot in dorsiflexion and strike the Achilles tendon directly (Fig. 16.13). Feel the normal response as the foot plantar flexes against your hand.

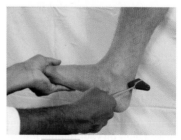

16.13 Achilles reflex.

Normal Range of Findings	**Abnormal Findings**

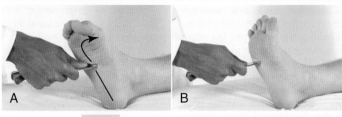

16.14   (A) Plantar reflex. (B) Babinski sign.

Plantar Reflex (L4 to S2). Position the thigh in slight external rotation. With the reflex hammer, draw a light stroke up the lateral side of the sole of the foot and inward across the ball of the foot, like an upside-down J shape (Fig. 16.14, *A*). The normal response is plantar flexion of the toes and inversion and flexion of the forefoot.

Except in infancy, the abnormal response is dorsiflexion of the big toe and fanning of all toes, which is a **positive Babinski sign**, also called *upgoing toes* (Fig. 16.14, *B*). This occurs with upper motor neuron disease of the corticospinal (or pyramidal) tract.

❖ DEVELOPMENTAL CONSIDERATIONS

Infants (Birth to 12 Months)

Assessment includes noting that milestones you normally would expect for each month have indeed been achieved and that the early, more primitive reflexes are eliminated from the baby's repertory when they are supposed to be.

Failure to attain a skill by expected time.

Persistence of reflex behaviour beyond the normal time.

The Motor System. Observe spontaneous motor activity for smoothness and symmetry. Smoothness of movement suggests proper cerebellar function, as does the coordination involved in sucking and swallowing. To screen gross and fine motor coordination, use the Nipissing District Developmental Screen (NDDS), or other parent-report screening tool. (See pages 24–25 in Jarvis, *Physical Examination and Health Assessment*, 3rd Canadian edition, for more information.)

Delay in motor activity occurs with brain damage, intellectual disability, peripheral neuromuscular damage, prolonged illness, and parental neglect.

Continued

Normal Range of Findings	Abnormal Findings

Check the muscle tone necessary for head control. With the baby supine and holding the wrists, pull the infant into a sitting position and note head control. The newborn will hold the head in almost the same plane as the body, and the head will balance briefly when the baby reaches a sitting position, then flop forward. (Even a premature infant shows some head flexion.) At 4 months of age, the head stays in line with the body and does not flop.

Because development progresses in a cephalocaudal direction, head lag is an early sign of brain damage.

Any baby who cannot hold the head in midline when sitting after 6 months of age should be referred for neurological evaluation.

Infantile automatisms are reflexes that have a predictable timetable of appearance and disappearance. For the screening examination, check the rooting, grasp (palmar and plantar), tonic neck, and Moro reflexes.

Rooting Reflex. Brush the infant's cheek near the mouth. The infant normally turns the head toward that side and opens the mouth. The reflex appears at birth and disappears within 3 or 4 months.

Palmar Grasp. Offer your finger from the baby's ulnar side, away from the thumb, and note tight grasp of all the baby's fingers. Sucking enhances grasp. You can often pull baby to a sit with the palmar grasp. The reflex is present at birth, is strongest at 1 to 2 months, and disappears at 3 to 4 months.

The palmar grasp reflex is absent with brain damage and with local muscle or nerve injury.

The palmar grasp reflex persists after 4 months of age with frontal lobe lesion.

Plantar Grasp. Touch your thumb at the ball of the baby's foot. Note that the toes curl down tightly. This reflex is present at birth and disappears at 8 to 10 months.

Babinski Reflex. Stroke your finger up the lateral edge and across the ball of the infant's foot. Note fanning of toes (positive Babinski reflex; Fig. 16.15). The reflex is present at birth and disappears (changes to the adult response) by 24 months of age (variable).

The Babinski reflex persists after 2 or 2½ years of age with pyramidal tract disease.

Normal Range of Findings	Abnormal Findings

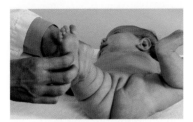

16.15 Babinski reflex.

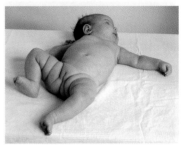

16.16 Tonic neck reflex.

Tonic Neck Reflex. With the baby supine, relaxed, or sleeping, turn the head to one side with the chin over the shoulder. Note ipsilateral extension of the arm and leg and flexion of the opposite arm and leg; this is the "fencing" position. If you turn the infant's head to the opposite side, arm and leg positions will reverse (Fig. 16.16). The reflex appears by 2 to 3 months, decreases at 3 to 4 months, and disappears by 4 to 6 months.

Moro Reflex. Startle the infant by jarring the crib, making a loud noise, or supporting the head and back in a semi-sitting position and quickly lowering the infant to 30 degrees. The baby looks as if he or she is hugging a tree; that is, there is symmetrical abduction and extension of the arms and legs, fanning of fingers, and curling of the index finger and thumb to a C-shape position. The infant then brings in both arms and legs (Fig. 16.17). The reflex is present at birth and disappears at 1 to 4 months.

Persistence later in infancy occurs with brain damage.

Absence of the Moro reflex in the newborn or persistence after 5 months of age indicates severe CNS injury.

Absence of movement in one arm occurs with fracture of the humerus or clavicle and with brachial nerve palsy.

Absence of movement in one leg occurs with a lower spinal cord problem or a dislocated hip.

A hyperactive Moro reflex appears hyperactive with tetany or CNS infection.

Older Adults

Use the same examination as used with younger adults. Be aware that some older adults show a slower response to your requests, especially to those calling for coordination of movements.

Continued

Normal Range of Findings	Abnormal Findings

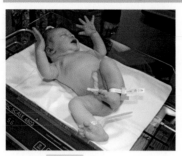

16.17 Moro reflex.

Any decrease in muscle bulk is most apparent in the hand, as seen by guttering between the metacarpals. These dorsal hand muscles often look wasted, even with no apparent arthropathy. The grip strength remains relatively good.

Senile tremors occasionally occur. These benign tremors include an intention tremor of the hands, head nodding (as if saying yes or no), and tongue protrusion. *Dyskinesias* are the repetitive stereotyped movements in the jaw, lips, or tongue that may accompany senile tremors (see Table 16.1). There is no associated rigidity.

The gait may be slower, may be more deliberate, and may deviate slightly from a midline path compared with the gait in the younger person.

After 65 years of age, loss of the sensation of vibration at the ankle malleolus is common and is usually accompanied by loss of the ankle jerk. Tactile sensation may be impaired. The older adult may need stronger stimuli for light touch and especially pain.

The deep tendon reflexes (DTRs) are less brisk. Those in the upper extremities are usually present, but the ankle jerks are commonly lost. Knee jerks may be lost, but this occurs less often.

Hand muscle atrophy is worsened with disuse and degenerative arthropathy.

Distinguish senile tremors from tremors of parkinsonism. The latter includes rigidity, slowness, and weakness of voluntary movement.

Absence of a rhythmic, reciprocal gait pattern is seen in parkinsonism and hemiparesis.

Note any difference in sensation between the right and left sides, which may indicate a neurological deficit.

Normal Range of Findings	Abnormal Findings

The plantar reflex may be absent or difficult to interpret. Often you will not see a definite normal flexor response; however, you should still consider a definite extensor response to be abnormal.

Neurological Recheck

Some hospitalized patients have a neurological deficit caused by head trauma or a systemic disease process. These patients must be monitored closely for any improvement or deterioration in neurological status and for any indication of increasing intracranial pressure.

Conduct an abbreviated neurological examination in the following sequence:
1. Level of consciousness
2. Motor function
3. Pupillary response
4. Vital signs

Level of Consciousness. A *change* in the level of consciousness is the single most important factor in this examination. It is the earliest and most sensitive index of change in neurological status. Note the ease of *arousal* and the state of awareness, or *orientation*. Assess orientation by asking questions about the following:
• Person: own name, occupation, names of workers around person, their occupations
• Place: where person is, nature of building, city, province
• Time: day of week, month, year

Vary the questions during repeat assessments so that the patient is not merely memorizing answers.

Note the quality and content of the verbal response, as well as articulation, fluency, manner of thinking, and any deficit in language comprehension or production (see Chapter 2, page 12).

A change in consciousness may be subtle. Note any decreasing level of consciousness, disorientation, memory loss, uncooperative behaviour, or even complacency in a previously combative patient.

Continued

Normal Range of Findings	Abnormal Findings
A patient is fully alert when his or her eyes open at your approach or spontaneously; when he or she is oriented to person, place, and time; and when he or she is able to follow verbal commands appropriately.	Review Table 2.1, Levels of Consciousness, Chapter 2, p. 13.

If the patient is not fully alert, increase the amount of stimulus used in this order:
1. Name called
2. Light touch on patient's arm
3. Vigorous shake of patient's shoulder
4. Pain applied (pinch the patient's nail bed or pinch trapezius muscle; rub your knuckles on the patient's sternum)

Record the stimulus used as well as the patient's response to it.

Motor Function. Check the voluntary movement of each extremity by giving the patient specific commands. (This procedure also tests level of consciousness by noting the patient's ability to follow commands.)

Ask the patient to lift the eyebrows, frown, and bare the teeth. Note symmetrical facial movements and bilateral nasolabial folds (cranial nerve VII).

Check upper arm strength by checking hand grasps. Ask the patient to squeeze your fingers. Offer your two fingers, one on top of the other, so that a strong hand grasp does not hurt your knuckles.

Check lower extremities by asking the patient to do straight leg raises. Ask the supine patient to lift one leg at a time straight up off the bed. Full strength allows the leg to be lifted 90 degrees. If multiple trauma, pain, or equipment precludes this motion, ask the patient to push one foot at a time against your hand's resistance, "like putting your foot on the gas pedal of your car."

Normal Range of Findings	Abnormal Findings

For the patient with decreased level of consciousness, note if movement occurs spontaneously as a result of noxious stimuli, such as pain or suctioning. An attempt to push away your hand after such stimuli is called *localizing* and is characterized as purposeful movement.

Any abnormal posturing, decorticate rigidity, or decerebrate rigidity indicates diffuse brain injury. (See Table 25.9, p. 744, in Jarvis: *Physical* Examination and Health Assessment, 3rd Canadian edition.)

Pupillary Response. Note the size, shape, and symmetry of both pupils. Shine a light into each pupil and note the direct and consensual light reflex. Both pupils should constrict briskly. (Allow for the effects of any medication that could affect pupil size and reactivity.) When recording, pupil size is best expressed in millimetres. Tape a millimetre scale onto a tongue blade and hold it next to the patient's eyes for the most accurate measurement (Fig. 16.18).

In a brain-injured patient, a sudden, unilateral, dilated, and nonreactive pupil is an ominous sign. Cranial nerve III runs parallel to the brain stem. When increasing intracranial pressure pushes the brain stem down (uncal herniation), it puts pressure on cranial nerve III, causing pupil dilation.

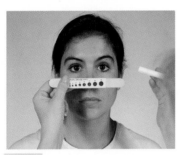

16.18   Measure pupil size in millimetres.

Vital Signs. Measure the temperature, pulse, respiration, and blood pressure as often as the patient's condition warrants. Although they are vital to the overall assessment of the critically ill patient, pulse and blood pressure are notoriously unreliable parameters of CNS deficit. Any changes are late consequences of rising intracranial pressure.

The *Cushing reflex* consists of signs of increasing intracranial pressure: sudden elevation of blood pressure with widening pulse pressure and decreased pulse rate or slow and bounding pulse.

Continued

Normal Range of Findings	Abnormal Findings

Assessment of Unconscious and Brain-Damaged Patients

The Glasgow Coma Scale

The assessment of *comatose* patients is an important aspect of critical care. The Glasgow Coma Scale (Fig. 16.19) was originally designed for patients with head trauma and has become the most widely used scoring system for patients with an altered level of consciousness in the critical care unit (Fischer et al., 2010). The GCS is used to assess the functional state of the brain as a whole, not of any particular site in the brain, and it is a standardized assessment that defines the level of consciousness by giving it a numerical value.

  The scale is divided into three areas: eye opening, motor response, and verbal response. Each area is rated separately, and a number is given for the patient's best response. The three numbers are added; the total score reflects the brain's functional level. A fully alert, normal patient has a score of 15. Serial assessments can be plotted on a graph to illustrate visually whether the patient is stable, improving, or deteriorating.

A score of 7 or less reflects coma.

The Canadian Neurological Scale

This valid, reliable, and standard neurological assessment tool is used to evaluate and monitor both mentation (level of consciousness, orientation, and speech) and motor function (face, arm, and leg) in patients with stroke. (See Fig. 25.61, page 732, in Jarvis: *Physical Examination & Health Assessment*, 3rd Canadian edition.)

16.19 Glasgow Coma Scale. (*Images © Pat Thomas, 2014.*)

Summary Checklist: Neurological Examination

Screening Neurological Examination

1. **Mental status**
2. **Cranial nerves**
   II: Optic
   III, IV, VI: Extraocular muscles
   V: Trigeminal
   VII: Facial mobility
3. **Motor function**
   Gait and balance
   Knee flexion: hop or shallow
      knee bend
4. **Sensory function**
   Superficial pain and light touch:
      arms and legs
   Vibration: arms and legs
5. **Reflexes**
   Biceps
   Triceps
   Patellar
   Achilles

Complete Neurological Examination

1. **Mental status**
2. **Cranial nerves II through XII**
3. **Motor system**
   Muscle size, strength, tone
   Gait and balance
   Rapid alternating movements
4. **Sensory function**
   Superficial pain and light touch
   Vibration
   Position sense
   Stereognosis, graphesthesia, two-
      point discrimination
5. **Reflexes**
   Deep tendon: biceps, triceps,
      brachioradialis, patellar,
      Achilles
   Superficial: abdominal, plantar

ABNORMAL FINDINGS

| TABLE 16.1 | Abnormalities in Muscle Movement |

Paralysis

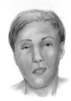

Decrease in, or loss of, motor power caused by problem with motor nerve or muscle fibres. Acute causes: trauma, spinal cord injury, cerebrovascular accident, poliomyelitis, polyneuritis, Bell's palsy; chronic causes: muscular dystrophy, diabetic neuropathy, multiple sclerosis; episodic causes: myasthenia gravis.

Patterns of paralysis: *hemiplegia* (spastic or flaccid paralysis of one [right or left] side of body and extremities); *paraplegia* (symmetrical paralysis of both lower extremities); *quadriplegia* (paralysis in all four extremities); *paresis* (weakness of muscles rather than paralysis).

Tic

Involuntary, compulsive, repetitive twitching of a muscle group such as wink, grimace, head movement, shoulder shrug; has a neurological cause such as tardive dyskinesias or Tourette's syndrome, or psychogenic cause (habit tic).

Fasciculation

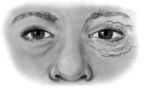

Rapid, continuous twitching of resting muscle or part of muscle, without movement of limb, which can be seen or palpated. Types: fine (occurs with lower motor neuron disease, associated with atrophy and weakness); coarse (occurs with cold exposure or fatigue and is not significant).

Myoclonus

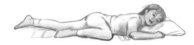

Rapid, sudden jerk or short series of jerks at fairly regular intervals. A hiccup is a myoclonus of the diaphragm. Single myoclonic arm or leg jerk is normal when a person is falling asleep; myoclonic jerks are severe with grand mal seizures.

Continued

TABLE 16.1	Abnormalities in Muscle Movement—cont'd

Tremor

Involuntary contraction of opposing muscle groups. Results in rhythmic, back-and-forth movement of one or more joints. May occur at rest or with voluntary movement. All tremors disappear during sleep. Tremors may be slow (3–6 per second) or rapid (10–20 per second).

Rest Tremor

Coarse and slow (3–6 per second); partly or completely disappears with voluntary movement (e.g., "pill rolling" tremor of parkinsonism, with thumb and opposing fingers).

Intention Tremor

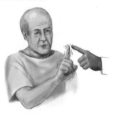

Rate varies; worse with voluntary movement. Occurs with cerebellar disease and multiple sclerosis. Essential tremor (familial): a type of intention tremor; most common tremor with older people. Benign (no associated disease), but causes emotional stress in work or social situations. Improves with the administration of sedatives, propranolol, and alcohol, but use of alcohol is discouraged because of the risk for addiction.

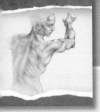

CHAPTER 17

Male Genitourinary System

STRUCTURE AND FUNCTION

The male genital structures include the penis and scrotum externally, and the testis, epididymis, and vas deferens internally (Fig. 17.1). The accessory glandular structures (prostate, seminal vesicles, and bulbourethral glands) are discussed in Chapter 19.

The **urethra** traverses the corpus spongiosum, and its meatus forms a slit at the glans tip.

The **scrotum** is a loose protective sac that is a continuation of the abdominal wall. In each scrotal half is a **testis,** which produces sperm. The testis has a solid oval structure and is about 4 to 5 cm long by 3 cm wide in adults.

The testis is capped by the **epididymis,** which is a markedly coiled duct system that is the main storage site of sperm. The epididymis is continuous with a muscular duct, the **vas deferens,** which approximates with other vessels to form the **spermatic cord.** The spermatic cord runs through the inguinal canal into the abdomen.

Puberty begins sometime between the ages of 9½ and 13½. The first sign is enlargement of the testes. Next, pubic hair appears, and then penis size increases. The stages of development are documented in

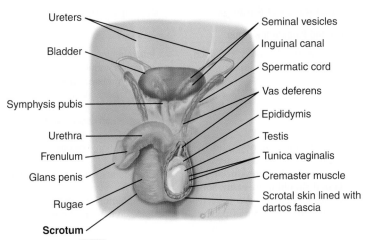

Ureters	Seminal vesicles
Bladder	Inguinal canal
	Spermatic cord
	Vas deferens
Symphysis pubis	Epididymis
Urethra	Testis
Frenulum	Tunica vaginalis
Glans penis	Cremaster muscle
Rugae	Scrotal skin lined with dartos fascia
Scrotum	

17.1 Male genital structures. *(© Pat Thomas, 2010.)*

Tanner's sexual maturity rating. See Table 26.1, p. 751, in Jarvis: *Physical Examination and Health Assessment,* 3rd Canadian edition.

The complete change in male genitalia development from preadolescent to adult takes about 3 years; the normal range is 2 to 5 years.

SUBJECTIVE DATA

1. Frequency, urgency, and nocturia
2. Dysuria (pain or burning with urination)
3. Hesitancy and straining
4. Urine colour (cloudy or hematuria)
5. Genitourinary history (kidney disease, kidney stones, flank pain, urinary tract infections, prostate trouble)
6. Penis: pain, lesion, discharge
7. Scrotum: self-care behaviours; lumps or swelling
8. Sexual activity and contraceptive use
9. Sexually transmitted infection (STI) contact

OBJECTIVE DATA

PREPARATION

Position the male standing with undershorts down and appropriate draping. The examiner should be sitting. Alternatively, the male may be supine for the first part of the examination and then stand during the hernia check.

EQUIPMENT NEEDED

Gloves: Wear gloves during every male genitalia examination
Glass slide for urethral specimen (occasionally)
Materials for cytological study
Flashlight

Normal Range of Findings	Abnormal Findings
Inspect and Palpate the Penis	
The skin normally looks wrinkled, hairless, and without lesions.	Inflammation. Lesions: nodules, solitary ulcer (chancre), grouped vesicles or superficial ulcers, wartlike papules (see Table 26.4, p. 770, in Jarvis: *Physical Examination and Health Assessment,* 3rd Canadian edition.).
The glans looks smooth and free of lesions. Ask the uncircumcised male to retract the foreskin, or you retract it. It should move easily. Some cheesy smegma may have collected under the foreskin. After inspection, slide the foreskin back to the original position.	Inflammation; lesions on glans or corona. **Phimosis:** inability to retract the foreskin **Paraphimosis:** inability to return the foreskin to original position.

Normal Range of Findings	Abnormal Findings
The urethral meatus is positioned just about centrally on the glans.	**Hypospadias:** ventral location of meatus.
	Epispadias: dorsal location of meatus (see Table 26.5, p. 773, in Jarvis: *Physical Examination and Health Assessment,* 3rd Canadian edition.).
Compress the glans anteroposteriorly between your thumb and forefinger. The edge of the meatus should appear pink, smooth, and without discharge.	Stricture: narrowed opening.
	Edges that are red, everted, and edematous, along with purulent discharge, suggest urethritis. (See Table 26.3, p. 769, in Jarvis: *Physical Examination and Health Assessment,* 3rd Canadian edition.)
Palpate the shaft between your thumb and first two fingers. The penis normally feels smooth, semi-firm, and nontender.	Nodule or induration. Tenderness.

Inspect and Palpate the Scrotum

Scrotal size varies with ambient room temperature. Asymmetry is normal, with the left scrotal half usually lower than the right. Lift the sac to inspect the posterior surface. Normally, there are no scrotal lesions except for the commonly found sebaceous cysts. These are yellowish, 1-cm nodules that are firm, nontender, and often multiple.	Scrotal swelling (edema) may be taut and pitting. This occurs with heart failure, renal failure, and local inflammation. Lesions should be investigated. Inflammation.
Gently palpate each scrotal half between your thumb and first two fingers. Testes normally feel oval, firm and rubbery, and smooth and equal bilaterally. They are freely movable and slightly tender to moderate pressure. Each epididymis normally feels discrete, softer than the testis, smooth, and nontender.	Absence of testis: may be a temporary migration or true cryptorchidism (Table 17.1). Atrophied testes—small and soft. Fixed testes. Nodules on testes or epididymides. Marked tenderness. An indurated, swollen, and tender epididymis: indicative of epididymitis. Thickened cord.
Between your thumb and forefinger, palpate each spermatic cord along its length, from the epididymis up to the external inguinal ring. You should feel a smooth and nontender cord.	Soft, swollen, and tortuous cord (see varicocele, Table 17.1).

Continued

Normal Range of Findings

Normally, there are no other scrotal contents. If you do find a mass, note the following:

- Is there any tenderness?
- Is the mass distal or proximal to the testis?
- Can you place your fingers over it?
- Does it reduce when the patient lies down?
- Can you auscultate bowel sounds over it?

Inspect and Palpate for Hernia

Inspect the inguinal region for a bulge as the patient stands and as he strains down. Normally none is present.

Palpate the inguinal canal (Fig. 17.2). Ask the patient to shift his weight onto the left (unexamined) leg. Place your right index finger low on the right scrotal half. Palpate up the length of the spermatic cord, invaginating the scrotal skin as you go, to the external inguinal ring. The inguinal ring feels like a triangular, slitlike opening, and it may or may not admit your finger. If it will admit your finger, gently insert it into the canal and ask the patient to "bear down." Normally, you will feel no change. Repeat the procedure on the left side.

Palpate the femoral area for a bulge. Normally, you feel none.

Abnormal Findings

Abnormalities in the scrotum: hernia, tumour, orchitis, epididymitis, hydrocele, spermatocele, varicocele (see Table 17.1).

Bulge at external inguinal ring or femoral canal should be investigated. (A hernia may be present but is easily reduced and may appear only intermittently with an increase in intra-abdominal pressure.)

A palpable herniating mass bumps your fingertip or pushes against the side of your finger. (See Table 26.7, p. 777, in Jarvis: *Physical Examination and Health Assessment,* 3rd Canadian edition.)

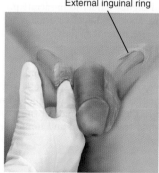

External inguinal ring

17.2 Palpate for inguinal hernia.

Normal Range of Findings	Abnormal Findings

Palpate Inguinal Lymph Nodes

Palpate the horizontal chain along the groin inferior to the inguinal ligament and the vertical chain along the upper inner thigh.

On occasion, it is normal to palpate an isolated node. It feels small (<1 cm), soft, discrete, and movable.

Enlarged, hard, matted, fixed nodes.

Self-Care: Testicular Self-Examination (TSE)

The incidence of testicular cancer is rare, but most commonly occurs in men ages 15 to 29. Encourage self-care by teaching each male 15 years and older to be aware of the normal look and feel of his testicles.

A testicular tumour has no early symptoms. If it is detected early by palpation and treated, the cure rate is almost 100%.

A good time to examine the testicles is just after a warm bath or shower. The heat from the water relaxes the scrotum and makes the testicles descend. Carefully feel each testicle for any changes such as a lump or tenderness. The testicle is egg-shaped and movable. It feels rubbery with a smooth surface, like a peeled hard-boiled egg. The epididymis is a tube on top and behind each testicle; it feels like a soft cord or a small bump. Report any changes to a doctor as soon as possible (Canadian Cancer Society, 2017b).

❖ DEVELOPMENTAL CONSIDERATIONS

Infants and Children

Palpate the scrotum and testes. Take care not to elicit the cremasteric reflex that pulls the testes up into the inguinal canal; keep your hands warm and palpate from the external inguinal ring down, and block the inguinal canals with the thumb and forefinger of your other hand to prevent the testes from retracting (Fig. 17.3).

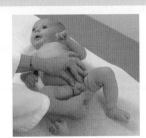

17.3 Palpate infant testes.

Continued

Normal Range of Findings	Abnormal Findings
Normally, the testes are descended and are equal in size bilaterally (1.5 to 2 cm until puberty). Once palpated, testes are considered descended, even if they have retracted momentarily at the next visit. If the scrotal half feels empty, search for the testes along the inguinal canal and try to milk them down. Ask the toddler or child to squat with the knees flexed up: this pressure may force the testes down. Another manoeuvre is to have the young child sit cross-legged to relax the reflex. Migratory testes (physiological cryptorchidism) are common because of the strength of the cremasteric reflex and the small mass of the prepubertal testes. Note that the affected side has a normally developed scrotum and that the testis can be milked down. These testes descend at puberty and are normal.	**Cryptorchidism:** undescended testes (those that have never descended). Undescended testes are common in premature infants. They occur in 3 to 4% of term infants, although most have descended by 3 months of age. Physicians have different opinions concerning the age at which an affected child should be referred (Table 17.1). With true cryptorchidism, the scrotum is atrophic.

Older Adults

In the older male, you may note thinner, greying pubic hair and decreased size of the penis. Testes may decrease in size and feel less firm. The scrotal sac is pendulous, with fewer rugae. The scrotal skin may become excoriated if the man continually sits on it.

Summary Checklist: Male Genitalia Examination

1. **Inspect** and **palpate** the **penis**
2. **Inspect** and **palpate** the **scrotum**
3. **If a mass exists,** transilluminate the scrotum
4. **Palpate** for an **inguinal hernia**
5. **Palpate** the **inguinal lymph nodes**
6. **Engage in teaching and health promotion**

ABNORMAL FINDINGS

TABLE 17.1	Abnormalities in the Scrotum	
Disorder	Clinical Findings	Discussion
Absent Testis (Cryptorchidism)	S: Empty scrotal half. O: Inspection: in true maldescent, atrophic scrotum on affected side. Palpation: no testis. A: Absence of testis.	True cryptorchidism: testes that have never descended. Incidence at birth is 3%–4%: one-half of these descend in first month. Incidence with premature infants is 30%; in the adult, 0.7%–0.8%. True undescended testes have a histological change by 6 years, causing decreased spermatogenesis and infertility.
Small Testis	S: None. O: Palpation: small and soft (rarely may be firm). A: Small testis.	Smallness with softness (<3.5 cm) indicates atrophy as with cirrhosis, hypopituitarism, after estrogen therapy, or as a sequela of orchitis. Smallness with firmness (<2 cm) occurs with Klinefelter's syndrome (hypogonadism).
Testicular Torsion 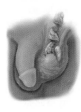	S: Excruciating pain in testicle, of sudden onset, often during sleep or after trauma. May also have lower abdominal pain, nausea and vomiting, no fever. O: Inspection: red, swollen scrotum, one testis (usually left) higher as a result of rotation and shortening. Palpation: cord feels thick, swollen, tender; epididymis may be anterior; cremasteric reflex is absent on side of torsion. A: Acute, painful swelling of spermatic cord, with elevation of one testis.	Sudden twisting of spermatic cord. Occurs in late childhood and early adolescence, rare after age 20 years. Torsion occurs usually on the left side. Faulty anchoring of testis on wall of scrotum allows testis to rotate. The anterior part of the testis rotates medially toward the other testis. Blood supply is cut off, resulting in ischemia and engorgement. This is an emergency requiring surgery; testis can become gangrenous in a few hours.

Continued

TABLE 17.1	Abnormalities in the Scrotum—cont'd	
Disorder	**Clinical Findings**	**Discussion**
Epididymitis 	S: Severe pain of sudden onset in scrotum, somewhat relieved by elevation (a positive Phren sign); also rapid swelling, fever. O: Inspection: enlarged scrotum; reddened. Palpation: exquisitely tender; epididymis enlarged, indurated; may be hard to distinguish from testis. Overlying scrotal skin may be thick and edematous. Laboratory: white blood cells and bacteria in urine. A: Tender swelling of epididymis.	Acute infection of epididymis commonly caused by prostatitis; occurs after prostatectomy because of trauma of urethral instrumentation, or due to *Chlamydia*, gonorrhea, or other bacterial infection. Often difficult to distinguish between epididymitis and testicular torsion.
Varicocele 	S: Dull pain; constant pulling or dragging sensation; or may be asymptomatic. O: Inspection: usually no sign. May show bluish colour through light scrotal skin. Palpation: when patient is standing, a soft, irregular mass is palpable posterior to and above testis; collapses when supine, refills when upright. Feels distinctive, like a "bag of worms." The testis on the side of the varicocele may be smaller owing to impaired circulation. A: Soft mass on spermatic cord.	A varicocele is a collection of dilated, tortuous varicose veins in the spermatic cord as a result of incompetent valves within the vein, which enable reflux of blood. Most often on left side, perhaps because left spermatic vein is longer and inserts at a right angle into left renal vein. Common in boys and young men. Screen at early adolescence; early treatment important to prevent potential infertility in adulthood.
Spermatocele 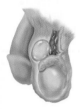	S: Painless, usually found on examination. O: Inspection: can be transilluminated higher in the scrotum than a hydrocele, and the sperm may be fluorescent. Palpation: round, freely movable mass lying above and behind testis. If large, feels like a third testis. A: Free cystic mass on epididymis.	Retention cyst in epididymis. Cause unclear but may be obstruction of tubules. Filled with thin, milky fluid that contains sperm. Most spermatoceles are small (<1 cm); occasionally, they are larger and then may be mistaken for hydrocele.

TABLE 17.1	Abnormalities in the Scrotum—cont'd	
Disorder	**Clinical Findings**	**Discussion**
Early Testicular Tumour	S: Painless, found on examination. O: Palpation: firm nodule or harder than normal section of testicle. A: Solitary nodule.	Most testicular tumours occur in men between the ages of 15 and 29. Practically all are malignant and occur most often in men of European descent. Biopsy is necessary to confirm malignancy. Most important risk factor is undescended testis, even those surgically corrected. Early detection important in prognosis, but practice of testicular self-examination is currently low.
Diffuse Tumour	S: Enlarging testis (most common symptom). When enlarged, has feel of increased weight. O: Inspection: enlarged, cannot be transilluminated. Palpation: enlarged, smooth, ovoid, firm. Important: firm palpation does *not* cause usual sickening discomfort as with normal testis. A: Nontender swelling of testis.	Diffuse tumour maintains shape of testis.
Hydrocele	S: Painless swelling, although patient may complain of weight and bulk in scrotum. O: Inspection: enlarged; mass can be transilluminated, glows pink or red (in contrast to a hernia). Palpation: nontender mass, fingers can reach above mass (in contrast to scrotal hernia). A: Nontender swelling of testis.	Cystic. Circumscribed collection of serous fluid in tunica vaginalis, surrounding testis. May occur after epididymitis, trauma, hernia, tumour of testis, or spontaneously in a newborn.
Scrotal Hernia	S: Swelling; pain may occur with straining. O: Inspection: enlarged, may be reduced when patient is supine, cannot be transilluminated. Palpation: soft mushy mass; palpating fingers cannot reach above mass; mass is distinct from testicle that is normal. A: Nontender swelling of scrotum.	Scrotal hernia is usually a result of indirect inguinal hernia.

Continued

TABLE 17.1	Abnormalities in the Scrotum—cont'd	
Disorder	**Clinical Findings**	**Discussion**
Orchitis 	S: Acute or moderate pain of sudden onset, swollen testis, feeling of weight, fever. O: Inspection: enlarged, edematous, reddened; cannot be transilluminated. Palpation: swollen, congested, tense, and tender; hard to distinguish testis from epididymis. A: Tender swelling of testis.	Acute inflammation of testis. Most common cause is mumps; can occur with any infectious disease. May have associated hydrocele, which can be transilluminated.
Scrotal Edema	S: Tenderness. O: Inspection: enlarged, may be reddened (with local irritation). Palpation: taut with pitting; scrotal contents probably cannot be palpated. A: Scrotal edema.	Accompanies marked edema in lower half of body (e.g., in heart failure, renal failure, and portal vein obstruction). Occurs with local inflammation: epididymitis, torsion of spermatic cord. Also, obstruction of inguinal lymphatic vessels produces lymphedema of scrotum.

A, Assessment; *O,* objective data; *S,* subjective data.
Illustrations © Pat Thomas, 2006.

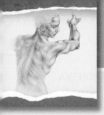

CHAPTER 18

Female Genitourinary System

STRUCTURE AND FUNCTION

EXTERNAL GENITALIA

The external female genitalia are called the **vulva,** or pudendum (Fig. 18.1). The **mons pubis** is a round, firm pad of adipose tissue covering the **symphysis pubis**. The **labia majora** and **labia minora** encircle a boat-shaped space, or cleft, termed the **vestibule.** Within this space, the **urethral meatus** appears as a dimple 2.5 cm posterior to the clitoris. The **clitoris** is a small, pea-shaped erectile body that is highly sensitive to tactile stimulation.

The **vaginal orifice** is posterior to the urethral meatus. On either side and posterior to the vaginal orifice are the two **vestibular (Bartholin's) glands,** which secrete a clear lubricating mucus during intercourse.

INTERNAL GENITALIA

The **vagina** is a flattened tubular canal extending from the orifice up and backward into the pelvis (Fig. 18.2). At

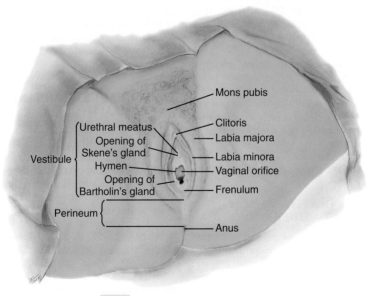

18.1 The external female genitalia.

237

ANTERIOR VIEW OF ADNEXA

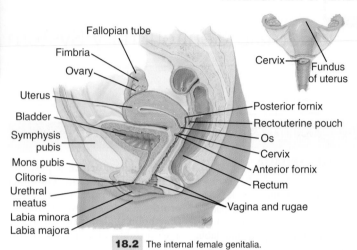

18.2 The internal female genitalia.

the end of the canal, the uterine **cervix** projects into the vagina.

The **uterus** is a pear-shaped, thick-walled, muscular organ. It is flattened anteroposteriorly, measuring 5.5 to 8 cm long by 3.5 to 4 cm wide and 2 to 2.5 cm thick. It is freely movable, not fixed, and usually tilts forward and superior to the bladder.

The **fallopian tubes** are two trumpet-shaped, pliable tubes, 10 cm in length, extending from the uterine fundus laterally to the brim of the pelvis, with their ends near the **ovaries**. Each ovary is oval, 3 cm long by 2 cm wide by 1 cm thick, and serves to develop ova (eggs), as well as the female hormones.

 DEVELOPMENTAL CONSIDERATIONS

The first signs of puberty are breast and pubic hair development, beginning between the ages of 8½ and 13 years. These signs are usually concurrent, but it is not abnormal if they do not develop together. They take about 3 years to complete.

Menarche occurs during the latter half of this sequence, just after the peak of growth velocity.

Irregularity of the menstrual cycle is common during adolescence because of occasional failure to ovulate. Tanner's table on the five stages of pubic hair development is helpful in teaching girls the expected sequence of sexual development (Table 18.1).

 SOCIAL DETERMINANTS OF HEALTH CONSIDERATIONS

Sexually transmitted infections (STIs) are a major health concern, with rates of chlamydia, gonorrhea, and infectious syphilis rising since the late 1990s. Chlamydia continues to be the most commonly reported STI in Canada; reported rates increased by 58% from 2003 to 2012 (Public Health Agency of Canada, 2015). Rates were highest in those aged 20 to 24 years, and women accounted for almost twice as many cases as did men. Some STIs are more common among lesbian and bisexual women, such as bacterial vaginosis, and are easily passed from woman to woman.

Urinary tract infection (UTI) is one of the most common bacterial infections in women (Epp & Larochelle, 2010). Women are more prone to developing UTIs than men because of the shortness of the female urethra, which makes it easier for bacteria to reach the bladder. Risk factors for development of UTI include abnormalities of the urinary tract, pregnancy, postmenopausal status, diabetes, and presence of an indwelling urinary catheter.

SUBJECTIVE DATA

1. Menstrual history
   - Last menstrual period (LMP)
   - Age at menarche
   - Cycle
   - Duration
   - Flow, clotting
   - Pain or cramps
2. Obstetrical history
   - Gravida: Number of pregnancies
   - Para: Number of births
   - Abortions: Interrupted pregnancies (elective abortions and spontaneous miscarriages)
3. Menopause
4. Self-care behaviours
   - Gynecological checkup, Pap smear
5. Urinary symptoms
   - Frequency, urgency
   - Dysuria, nocturia, hematuria
   - Incontinence (urgency or functional)
6. Vaginal discharge
   Colour, characteristics
7. Past history
8. Sexual activity
9. Contraceptive use
10. STI contact
11. STI risk reduction

OBJECTIVE DATA

PREPARATION

Initially, for the health history, the patient should be sitting up.

For the examination, the patient should be placed in the lithotomy position, with the examiner sitting on a stool. Help her into the lithotomy position, with the body supine, feet in stirrups and knees apart, and buttocks at edge of examining table. The arms should be at the patient's sides or across the chest, not over the head, because this position tightens the abdominal muscles.

Drape the patient fully, covering the stomach and legs, exposing only the vulva to your view. Be sure to push down the drape between the patient's legs, and elevate the head so that you can see her face.

EQUIPMENT NEEDED

Assemble these items before helping the patient into position. Arrange within easy reach.
Gloves
Goose-necked lamp with a strong light
Vaginal speculum of appropriate size
Graves speculum: useful for most women, available in varying lengths and widths
Pedersen speculum: narrow blades useful for young or postmenopausal women with a narrowed introitus
Large cotton-tipped applicators (rectal swabs)
Materials for cytological study:
   Glass slide with frosted end

You can help the patient relax, decrease her anxiety, and retain a sense of control by employing these measures:

- Have her empty the bladder before the examination.
- Position the examination table so that the perineum is not exposed to an inadvertent open door.
- Ask whether she would like a friend, family member, or chaperone present. Position this person by patient's head to maintain privacy.
- Elevate patient's head and shoulders to a semi-sitting position to maintain eye contact.
- Place the stirrups so the legs are not abducted too far.
- Explain each step in the examination before you do it.
- Assure the patient she can stop the examination at any point if she feels any discomfort.
- Use a gentle, firm touch and gradual movements.
- Maintain a dialogue throughout the examination to share information, answer questions, and provide health teaching.

Specimen container for liquid-based cytological study
Sterile Cytobrush or sterile cotton-tipped applicator
Ayre spatula
Spray fixative
Specimen container for gonorrhea/*Chlamydia* culture
Small bottle of normal saline solution, potassium hydroxide (KOH), and acetic acid (white vinegar)
Lubricant

Normal Range of Findings	Abnormal Findings
Inspect the External Genitalia	
Note the following characteristics:	
• Skin colour	
• Hair distribution is in the usual female pattern of inverted triangle, although it may normally trail up the abdomen toward the umbilicus.	Consider delayed puberty if no pubic hair or breast development has occurred by age 13 years.
	Nits or lice at the base of pubic hair.
• Labia majora are normally symmetrical, plump, and well formed. In nulliparous women, labia meet in the midline; following a vaginal delivery, the labia no longer meet in the midline, and appear slightly shrunken and less defined.	Swelling.

Normal Range of Findings	Abnormal Findings
• Skin texture: There should be no lesions, except for occasional sebaceous cysts. These are yellowish, 1-cm nodules that are firm, non-tender, and often multiple.	Excoriation, nodules, rash, or lesions. Refer any suspect pigmented lesion for evaluation and biopsy. (See Table 27.2, p. 809, in Jarvis: *Physical Examination and Health Assessment,* 3rd Canadian edition.)

With your gloved hand, separate the labia majora to inspect the following anatomical features:
- Clitoris.
- Labia minora are dark pink and moist, and usually symmetrical.
- Urethral opening appears stellate or slitlike and is midline.
- Vaginal opening, or introitus, may appear as a narrow vertical slit or as a larger opening.
- Perineum is smooth. A well-healed episiotomy scar, midline or mediolateral, may be present after a vaginal birth.
- Anus has coarse skin of increased pigmentation (see Chapter 19 for assessment).

Note that the following sections, which illustrate palpation of glands and examination of the internal female genitalia, are assessment approaches that go beyond the basic female genitourinary system assessment, and would normally be conducted only by an advanced practice nurse or physician.

Inflammation or lesions.

Polyp.

Foul-smelling, irritating discharge.

Palpate Glands

Assess urethra and Skene's glands. Dip your gloved finger in a bowl of warm water to lubricate. Insert your gloved index finger into the vagina, and gently milk the urethra by applying pressure up and out. This procedure should produce no pain. If any discharge appears, culture it.

Tenderness.
Induration along urethra.
Urethral discharge.

Assess Bartholin's glands. Palpate the posterior parts of the labia majora with your index finger in the vagina and your thumb outside (Fig. 18.3). The labia normally feel soft and homogeneous.

Swelling.
Pain with palpation.
Erythema around or discharge from duct opening.

Continued

Normal Range of Findings	Abnormal Findings

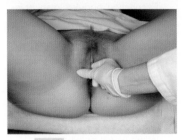

18.3 Palpate labia majora.

Assess the Support of Pelvic Musculature

- Palpate the perineum. It normally feels thick, smooth, and muscular in nulliparous women and thin and rigid in multiparous women.
- Using your index and middle fingers, separate the vaginal orifice and ask the woman to strain down. There is normally no bulging of vaginal walls or urinary incontinence.

Tenderness.
Paper-thin perineum.

Bulging of the vaginal wall indicates cystocele, rectocele, or uterine prolapse. (See Table 27.3, p. 811, in Jarvis: *Physical Examination and Health Assessment,* 3rd Canadian edition.)
Urinary incontinence should be investigated.

Internal Genitalia

Speculum Examination

Select the proper-sized speculum. Warm and lubricate the speculum under warm, running water. In many provinces, small amounts of carbomer-free, water-soluble lubricants are allowable for speculum exams for Papanicolaou (Pap) tests, as research indicates there is no effect on cervical cytology results (Lin et al., 2014).

Normal Range of Findings	Abnormal Findings

Hold the speculum in your left hand with the index and the middle fingers surrounding the blades and your thumb under the thumbscrew. This prevents the blades from opening painfully during insertion. With your right index and middle fingers, push the introitus down and open to relax the pubococcygeal muscle (Fig. 18.4).

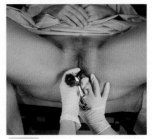

18.4 Invert vaginal speculum.

Tilt the width of the blades obliquely and insert the speculum past your right fingers, applying any pressure *downward*. This avoids pressure on the anterior vaginal wall and on the sensitive urethra above it.

Ease insertion by asking the patient to bear down. This method relaxes the perineal muscles and opens the introitus.

As the blades pass your right fingers, withdraw your fingers. Now change the hand holding the speculum to your right hand, and turn the width of the blades horizontally. Continue to insert in a 45-degree angle *downward* toward the small of the woman's back. This matches the natural slope of the vagina.

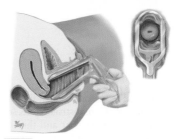

18.5 Open speculum blades and view cervix.

After the blades are fully inserted, open them by squeezing the handles together (Fig. 18.5). The cervix should be in full view. Lock the blades open by tightening the thumbscrew.

Inspect the Cervix and Its Os

Note the following characteristics:

- Colour. Normally, the cervical mucosa is pink and even. During the second month of pregnancy it looks blue (Chadwick's sign), and after menopause it is pale.

Redness, inflammation.
Pallor with anemia.
Cyanosis other than with pregnancy.
(See Table 27.4, p. 812, in Jarvis: *Physical Examination and Health Assessment,* 3rd Canadian edition.)

- Position. Midline, either anterior or posterior. It projects 1 to 3 cm into the vagina.

Lateral position may result from adhesion of tumour. Projection of more than 3 cm may be a prolapse.

Continued

Normal Range of Findings	Abnormal Findings
• Size. Diameter is 2.5 cm (1 inch).	Hypertrophy of more than 4 cm occurs with inflammation or tumour.
• Os. Small and round in nulliparous women. In parous women, it is a horizontal, irregular slit and may show healed lacerations on the sides.	
• Surface. Normally smooth, but **cervical eversion,** or ectropion, may occur normally after vaginal deliveries.	Reddened, granular, and asymmetrical surface, particularly around os. Friable, bleeding easily. Any lesions: white patch on cervix; strawberry spot. Refer any suspect red, white, or pigmented lesion for biopsy (see erosion, ulceration, and carcinoma, Table 27.4, p. 812, in Jarvis: *Physical Examination and Health Assessment,* 3rd Canadian edition).
• Cervical secretions. Depending on the day of the menstrual cycle, secretions may be clear and thin or thick, opaque, and stringy. They are always odourless and nonirritating.	Foul-smelling; irritating; or yellow, green, white, or grey discharge. (See Table 27.5, p. 813, in Jarvis: *Physical Examination and Health Assessment,* 3rd Canadian edition.)

If secretions are copious, swab the area with a thick-tipped rectal swab. This method sponges away secretions, giving you a better view of the structures.

Obtain Cervical Smears and Cultures

The Pap test is a screen for cervical cancer. Do not obtain a Pap test during the woman's menses or if a heavy infectious discharge is present. Instruct the woman not to douche, have intercourse, or put anything into the vagina within 24 hours before collecting the specimens. Conventional **glass slide cytology** remains the most common screening test for cervical cancer available in Canada. A single slide is sufficient for the entire specimen.

Normal Range of Findings	Abnormal Findings

Cervical Scrape. Insert the bifid end of a cervical spatula into the vagina, with the more pointed bump into the cervical os. Rotate it 360 to 720 degrees, using firm pressure (Fig. 18.6). The spatula scrapes the surface of the exocervix and the squamocolumnar junction (SCJ) or transformation zone (T-zone) as you turn the instrument. Spread the specimen from both sides of the spatula onto a glass slide. Use a single stroke to thin out the specimen, not a back-and-forth motion. Spray with a fixative (or not) according to your agency's procedures.

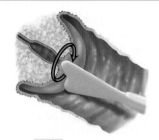

18.6 Cervical scrape.

Endocervical Specimen. Insert an endocervical brush into the os, and rotate it 720 degrees in *one* direction (Fig. 18.7). Then rotate the brush gently on a slide to deposit all the cells. Rotate in the opposite direction from the one in which you obtained the specimen. Avoid leaving a thick specimen that would be hard to read under the microscope. Immediately (within 2 seconds) spray the slide with fixative to avoid drying if procedures require this step.

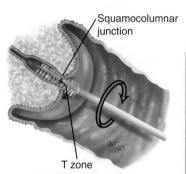

Squamocolumnar junction

T zone

18.7 Endocervical smear.

CAUTION: The endocervical brush is contraindicated for pregnant women.

Continued

Normal Range of Findings	Abnormal Findings

Inspect the Vaginal Wall

Loosen the thumbscrew, but continue to hold the speculum blades open. Slowly withdraw the speculum, rotating it as you go, to fully inspect the vaginal wall. Normally, the wall looks pink, deeply rugated, moist, and smooth, and it is free of inflammation or lesions. Normal discharge is thin and clear or opaque and stringy, but is always odourless.

When the blade ends near the vaginal opening, let them close, but be careful not to pinch the mucosa or catch any hairs. Turn the blades obliquely to avoid stretching the opening. Place the metal speculum in a basin to be cleaned later and soaked in a sterilizing and disinfecting solution; discard the plastic variety. Discard your gloves and wash hands.

Inflammation or lesions should be investigated.

Leukoplakia appears as a spot of dried white paint.

Vaginal discharge is abnormal when it has the following characteristics: thick, white, and curdlike (with candidiasis); profuse, watery, grey-green, and frothy (with trichomoniasis); or any grey, green-yellow, white, or foul-smelling discharge.

(See Table 27.5, p. 813, in Jarvis: *Physical Examination and Health Assessment,* 3rd Canadian edition.)

Bimanual Examination

Rise to a stand, and have the patient remain in the lithotomy position. Drop lubricant onto the first two fingers of the gloved hand that will be inserted intravaginally. Insert your lubricated fingers into the vagina, with any pressure directed posteriorly.

Use both hands to palpate the internal genitalia to assess their location, size, and mobility and to screen for any tenderness or mass. One hand is on the abdomen while the other (often the dominant, more sensitive hand) inserts two fingers into the vagina.

Palpate the Internal Genitalia

Palpate the vaginal wall. It normally feels smooth and has no area of induration or tenderness.

Nodule.
Tenderness.

Normal Range of Findings	Abnormal Findings

Locate the cervix in the midline, often near the anterior vaginal wall. Note the following characteristics of a normal cervix:

- Consistency: Feels smooth and firm, like the consistency of the tip of the nose. It softens and feels velvety at 5 to 6 weeks of pregnancy (Goodell's sign).

Hard with malignancy.
Nodular.

- Contour: Evenly rounded.
- Mobility: With a finger on either side, move the cervix gently from side to side. Normally this produces no pain (Fig. 18.8).

Irregular.
Immobile with malignancy.
Painful with inflammation or ectopic pregnancy.

Palpate all around the fornices; the wall should feel smooth.

Next, use your "abdominal" hand to push the pelvic organs closer for your intravaginal fingers to palpate. Place your hand midway between the umbilicus and the symphysis; push down in a slow, firm manner, with the fingers together and slightly flexed.

With your "intravaginal" fingers in the anterior fornix, assess the uterus. Determine the position, or *version,* of the uterus. In many women, the uterus is anteverted; you palpate it at the level of the pubis with the cervix pointing posteriorly. Two other positions normally occur (midposition and retroverted), as well as two aspects of flexion, where the long axis of the uterus is not straight but flexed (for illustration, see Fig. 27.19, page 802, in Jarvis: *Physical Examination and Health Assessment,* 3rd Canadian edition).

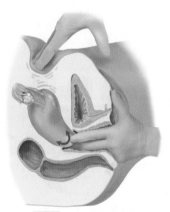

18.8 Palpate the cervix.

Palpate the uterine wall with your fingers in the fornices. It normally feels firm and smooth, with the contour of the fundus rounded. It softens during pregnancy. Bounce the uterus gently between your abdominal and intravaginal hands. It should be freely movable and nontender.

Enlarged uterus (see Table 27.6, p. 815, in Jarvis: *Physical Examination and Health Assessment,* 3rd Canadian edition).
Lateral displacement.
Nodular mass.
Irregular, asymmetrical uterus.
Fixed and immobile uterus.
Tenderness.

Continued

Normal Range of Findings	Abnormal Findings

Move both hands to the right to explore the adnexa. Place your abdominal hand on the lower quadrant just inside the anterior iliac spine with your intravaginal fingers in the lateral fornix (Fig. 18.9). Push the abdominal hand in and try to capture the ovary. In many patients, you cannot palpate the ovary. When you can, it normally feels smooth, firm, and almond-shaped; it is highly movable, sliding through the fingers. It is slightly sensitive but not painful. The fallopian tube is not normally palpable. No other mass or pulsation should be felt.

Enlarged adnexa; nodules or mass in adnexa.
   Immobile adnexa.
   Marked tenderness.

CRITICAL FINDING: Pulsation or a palpable fallopian tube suggests ectopic pregnancy and warrants immediate referral. (See Table 27.7, p. 816, in Jarvis; *Physical Examination and Health Assessment,* 3rd Canadian edition.)

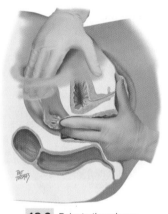

18.9   Palpate the adnexa.

Move to the left to palpate the other side. Then withdraw your hand and check secretions on the fingers before discarding the glove. Normal secretions are clear or cloudy and odourless.

A note of caution: Normal adnexal structures are often not palpable. To be safe, any mass that you cannot positively identify as a normal structure should be considered abnormal, and the woman should be referred for further study.

Normal Range of Findings	Abnormal Findings

Rectovaginal Examination

Use this technique to assess the recto-vaginal septum, posterior uterine wall, cul-de-sac, and rectum. Change gloves to avoid spreading any possible infection. Lubricate your first two fingers. Tell the woman this may feel uncomfortable and will mimic the feeling of moving her bowels. Ask her to bear down as you insert your index finger into the vagina and your middle finger gently into the rectum (Fig. 18.10).

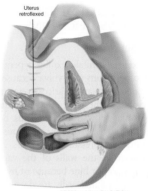

RECTOVAGINAL PALPATION

18.10

While pushing with the abdominal hand, repeat the steps of the bimanual examination. Try to keep the intravaginal finger on the cervix so the "intrarectal" finger does not mistake the cervix for a mass. Note the following characteristics:

- Rectovaginal septum should feel smooth, thin, firm, and pliable.
- Rectovaginal pouch, or cul-de-sac, is a potential space and usually not palpable.
- Uterine wall and fundus feel firm and smooth.

Rotate the intrarectal finger to check the rectal wall and anal sphincter tone. (See Chapter 19 for assessment of the anus and rectum.) Check your gloved finger as you withdraw it; test any adherent stool for occult blood.

Give the patient tissues to wipe the area and help her up. Remind her to slide her hips back from the table edge before sitting up so she does not fall.

Nodular or thickened.

Continued

Normal Range of Findings	Abnormal Findings

❖ DEVELOPMENTAL CONSIDERATIONS

Pregnant Women

The external genitalia exhibit hyperemia of the perineum and vulva because of increased vascularity. Varicose veins may be visible in the labia or legs. Hemorrhoids may show around the anus. Both are caused by interruption in venous return from the pressure of the fetus.

Internally, the walls of the vagina appear violet or blue because of hyperemia. The vaginal walls are deeply rugated, and the vaginal mucosa is thickened. The cervix looks blue and feels velvety and softer than in the nonpregnant state, making it a bit more difficult to differentiate from the vaginal walls.

During bimanual examination, the isthmus of the uterus feels softer and is more easily compressed between your two hands (Hegar's sign). The fundus balloons between your two hands; it feels connected to, but distinct from, the cervix because the isthmus is so soft.

Search the adnexal area carefully during early pregnancy. Normally, the adnexal structures are not palpable.

An ectopic pregnancy has serious consequences. (See Table 27.7, p. 816, in Jarvis: *Physical Examination and Health Assessment,* 3rd Canadian edition.)

Older Women

Natural lubrication is decreased; to avoid a painful examination, take care to lubricate instruments and the examining hand adequately. Use the Pedersen speculum (rather than the Graves) with its narrower, flatter blades.

Menopause and the resulting decrease in estrogen production cause numerous physical changes. Pubic hair gradually decreases, becoming thin and sparse in later years. The skin is thinner, and fat deposits decrease, leaving the mons pubis smaller and the labia flatter. Clitoris size also decreases after age 60 years.

Normal Range of Findings	Abnormal Findings
Internally, the rugae of the vaginal walls decrease, and the walls look pale pink because of the thinned epithelium. The cervix shrinks and looks pale and glistening. It may retract, appearing to be flush with the vaginal wall. In some older women, it is hard to distinguish the cervix from the surrounding vaginal mucosa. Alternately, the cervix may protrude into the vagina if the uterus has prolapsed. With the bimanual examination, the uterus feels smaller and firmer, and the ovaries are not normally palpable.	Refer any suspect red, white, or pigmented lesion for biopsy. Vaginal atrophy increases the risk for infection and trauma.

Summary Checklist: Female Genitalia Examination

1. **Inspect external genitalia**
2. **Palpate labia, Skene's,** and **Bartholin's glands**
3. Using vaginal speculum, **inspect cervix and vagina**
4. **Obtain specimens** for cytological study
5. **Perform bimanual examination:** cervix, uterus, adnexa
6. **Perform rectovaginal examination**
7. **Test stool** for occult blood
8. **Engage in teaching and health promotion**

ABNORMAL FINDINGS

TABLE 18.1	Sexual Maturity Rating in Girls	
Stage	Description	
1	Preadolescent. No pubic hair. Mons and labia covered with fine vellus hair, as on abdomen.	
2	Growth sparse and mostly on labia. Long, downy hair, slightly pigmented, straight or only slightly curly.	
3	Growth sparse and spreading over mons pubis. Hair is darker, coarser, and curlier.	
4	Hair is adult in type but over smaller area: none on medial thigh.	
5	Adult in type and pattern; inverse triangle. Also on medial thigh surface.	

Adapted from Tanner, J. M. (1962). *Growth at adolescence*. Oxford, England: Blackwell Scientific.

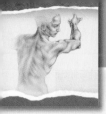

CHAPTER 19

Anus, Rectum, and Prostate

STRUCTURE AND FUNCTION

The **anal canal** is the outlet of the gastro-intestinal tract and is about 3.8 cm long in adults (Fig. 19.1). It slants forward toward the umbilicus, forming a distinct right angle with the rectum, which rests back in the hollow of the sacrum.

The anal canal is surrounded by two concentric layers of muscle: the *internal* and *external sphincters.*

The **rectum,** which is 12 cm long, is the distal portion of the large intestine. Just above the anal canal, the rectum dilates and turns posteriorly, forming the rectal ampulla.

In males, the **prostate gland** lies in front of the anterior wall of the rectum and 2 cm behind the symphysis pubis. It surrounds the bladder neck and the urethra, and it secretes a thin, milky alkaline fluid that helps sperm viability. It is a bilobed structure that is separated by a shallow groove called the **median sulcus.** The two **seminal vesicles** project like rabbit ears above the prostate. They secrete a fluid containing fructose, which nourishes the sperm.

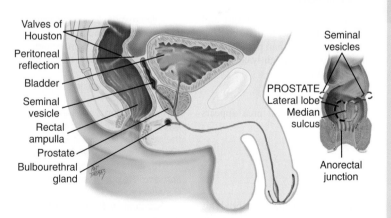

Valves of Houston
Peritoneal reflection
Bladder
Seminal vesicle
Rectal ampulla
Prostate
Bulbourethral gland

Seminal vesicles
PROSTATE
Lateral lobe
Median sulcus
Anorectal junction

19.1 Anatomy of the anal sphincters. (© *Pat Thomas, 2010.*)

SUBJECTIVE DATA

1. Usual bowel routine (frequency, stool colour, consistency)
2. Change in bowel habits (diarrhea, constipation)
3. Rectal bleeding, blood in the stool
4. Medications (laxatives, stool softeners, iron; use of enemas)
5. Rectal conditions (pruritus, hemorrhoids, fissure, fistula)
6. Family history (colon, rectal, prostate cancer; polyps; inflammatory bowel disease)
7. Self-care behaviours (diet of high-fibre foods, most recent examinations: **digital rectal examination [DRE]**, stool blood test, colonoscopy, **prostate-specific antigen [PSA]** blood test [for men])

OBJECTIVE DATA

PREPARATION

Examine the male patient in the left lateral decubitus position or standing position. Place the female patient in the lithotomy position if examining genitalia as well; use the left lateral decubitus position for examining the rectal area alone.

EQUIPMENT NEEDED

Penlight
Lubricating jelly
Glove
Guaiac test container

Normal Range of Findings	Abnormal Findings
Inspect the Perianal Area	
The anus normally looks moist and hairless, with coarse, folded skin that is more pigmented than perianal skin. The anal opening is tightly closed. No lesions are present.	Inflammation; lesions or scars. Linear split: fissure. Flabby skin sac: hemorrhoid. Shiny blue skin sac: thrombosed hemorrhoid. Small round opening in anal area: fistula.
The sacrococcygeal area appears smooth and even.	Inflammation or tenderness, swelling, a tuft of hair, or a dimple at the tip of the coccyx may indicate pilonidal cyst. (See Table 23.2, p. 619, in Jarvis: *Physical Examination and Health Assessment,* 3rd Canadian edition.)
Instruct the patient to hold his or her breath and bear down by performing a Valsalva's manoeuvre. There should be no break in skin integrity or protrusion through the anal opening.	Appearance of fissure or hemorrhoids. Circular red "doughnut" of tissue: rectal prolapse.

Normal Range of Findings	Abnormal Findings

Special Considerations for Advanced Practice

Palpate the Anus and Rectum

Drop lubricating jelly onto your gloved index finger. Inform the patient that palpation is not painful, but they may feel the need to move the bowels.

Place the pad of your index finger gently against the anal verge. You will feel the sphincter tighten, then relax. As it relaxes, flex the tip of your finger and slowly insert it into the anal canal in a direction toward the umbilicus.

Rotate your examining finger to palpate the entire muscular ring. The canal should feel smooth and even. To assess tone, ask the patient to tighten the muscle. The sphincter should tighten evenly around your finger without causing pain for the patient.

Decreased tone should be investigated.

Increased tone occurs with inflammation and anxiety.

Above the anal canal, the rectum turns posteriorly, following the curve of the coccyx and sacrum. Insert your finger farther and explore all around the rectal wall. It normally feels smooth with no nodularity. Promptly report any mass you discover for further examination.

An internal hemorrhoid above the anorectal junction is not palpable unless it is thrombosed.

A soft, slightly movable mass may be a polyp.

A firm or hard mass with irregular shape or rolled edges may signify carcinoma. (See Table 23.3, p. 622, in Jarvis: *Physical Examination and Health Assessment,* 3rd Canadian edition.)

In a female patient, palpate the cervix through the anterior rectal wall. It normally feels like a small round mass. You also may palpate a retroverted uterus or a tampon in the vagina. Do not mistake the cervix or a tampon for a tumour.

Continued

Normal Range of Findings	Abnormal Findings

Palpate the Prostate Gland

In male patients, palpate the prostate gland on the anterior wall (Fig. 19.2). Palpate the entire prostate in a systematic manner, but note that only the superior surface and part of the lateral surface are accessible to examination. Press *into* the gland at each location. Note these characteristics:

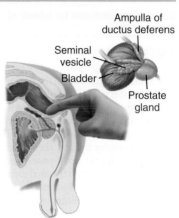

19.2 Palpating the prostate gland.

Size: 2.5 cm long by 4 cm wide; should not protrude more than 1 cm into the rectum

Shape: heart shape, with palpable central groove
Surface: smooth
Consistency: elastic, rubbery
Mobility: slightly movable
Sensitivity: nontender to palpation

In a transgender woman who has undergone vaginoplasty, the prostate remains in situ and may be palpated anteriorly via digital vaginal exam in a gender-affirming lithotomy position (Bournes, 2015).

Withdraw your examining finger; normally, there is no bright red blood or mucus on the glove. Offer the patient tissues to remove the lubricant, and help them to a more comfortable position.

Enlargement or atrophy.
Flatness with no groove.
Nodularity.
Hardness or boggy, soft, fluctuant texture.
Fixed position.
Tenderness.
Enlargement, firmness, and smoothness with central groove obliterated: suggestive of benign prostatic hypertrophy (BPH).
Swelling and exquisite tenderness: accompanies prostatitis.
Any stone-hard, irregular, fixed nodule indicates carcinoma. (See Table 23.4, p. 623, in Jarvis: *Physical Examination and Health Assessment,* 3rd Canadian edition.)

Normal Range of Findings	Abnormal Findings
Examination of Stool. Inspect any feces remaining on the glove. Normally, the colour is brown and the consistency is soft.	Jelly-like shreds of mucus mixed in stool indicate inflammation. Bright red blood on stool surface indicates rectal bleeding. Bright red blood mixed with feces indicates possible colonic bleeding.
Test any stool on the glove for **occult blood**. Use the specimen container that your agency directs. A negative response is normal. A positive *Hematest* indicates occult blood. However, a false-positive finding may occur if the patient has ingested significant amounts of red meat within 3 days of the test.	Black, tarry stool with distinct malodour indicates upper gastrointestinal bleeding, with blood partially digested. Black stool also occurs with ingesting iron medications or bismuth preparations. Grey, tan stool indicates the absence of bile pigment, as in obstructive jaundice. Pale yellow, greasy stool is indicative of increased fat content (steatorrhea), as occurs with malabsorption syndrome. Occult bleeding usually indicates cancer of colon.

Summary Checklist: Anus, Rectum, and Prostate Examination

1. **Inspect anus** and **perianal area**
2. **Inspect** during **Valsalva manoeuvre**
3. **Palpate anal canal** and **rectum** in all adults
4. **Test stool** for occult blood
5. **Engage in teaching and health promotion**

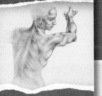

CHAPTER 20

The Complete Health Assessment: Putting It All Together

STRUCTURE AND FUNCTION

The following suggested examination sequence combines all the separate steps into a complete and smoothly flowing assessment. The sequence puts steps in clusters by body region, and proceeds systematically head to toe, concluding with examination of the genitalia. This is the most efficient way of conducting the examination, and it minimizes the number of position changes for you and the patient. The second column presents a sample recording when findings are within the normal range.

OBJECTIVE DATA

Sequence	Sample Recording
The patient walks into the room and sits; the examiner sits facing the patient; the patient remains in street clothes.	

The Health History

1. Collect the history, complete or limited as visit warrants. While obtaining the history and throughout the examination, note data on the patient's general appearance.

Continued

Sequence	Sample Recording

General Appearance

1. Appears stated age
2. Level of consciousness
3. Skin colour
4. Nutritional status
5. Posture and position comfortably erect
6. Obvious physical deformities
7. Mobility:
   Gait
   Use of assistive devices
   Range of motion (ROM) of joints
   Involuntary movements
   Ability to rise from a seated position
8. Facial expression
9. Mood and affect
10. Speech: articulation, pattern, content appropriate, first language
11. Hearing
12. Personal hygiene

(Patient's name) is a (age)-year-old (male/female), well nourished, well developed, who appears stated age. (S)he is alert, oriented, and cooperative, with no signs of acute distress. Appearance, behaviour, and speech are appropriate.

The following lined rules indicate position change for examiner or patient.

Measurement

1. Weight
2. Height
3. Calculate body mass index (BMI)
4. Waist and hip measurements (not indicated for patients younger than 18 years or for pregnant or lactating women)
5. Skinfold measurements (if indicated)
6. Vision using Snellen eye chart (if indicated)

Weight 57 kg (126 lb), height 163 cm (5'4"), waist 89 cm (35 inches), vision right eye 20/20, left eye 20/30—1.

Ask the patient to empty the bladder (save urine specimen, if needed), to disrobe except for underpants, and to put on a gown. The patient sits with the legs dangling off the side of the bed or table; examiner stands in front of the patient.

Sequence	Sample Recording

Skin

1. Examine both hands and inspect the nails.
2. For the rest of the examination, examine the skin of the corresponding region.

Skin colour tan-pink, warm to touch; turgor good, no lesions.
Nails: No clubbing or deformities, nail beds pink with prompt capillary refill.

Vital Signs

1. Radial pulse
2. Respirations
3. Blood pressure in arms
4. Blood pressure in lower leg; compute ankle/brachial index (if indicated)
5. Temperature (if indicated)
6. Oxygen saturation (if indicated)
7. Patient's rating of pain level on a scale of 0 to 10, note location of pain (use FACES Pain Rating Scale if appropriate).

TPR: 37°C–76–14, BP 128/84 right arm, sitting.
Reports no areas of pain.

Head and Face

1. Inspect and palpate scalp, hair, and cranium.
2. Inspect face: expression, symmetry (cranial nerve VII).
3. Palpate the temporal artery and then the temporomandibular joint as the patient opens and closes the mouth.
4. Palpate the maxillary sinuses and the frontal sinuses.

Hair: Texture fine, distribution appropriate for age.
Head: Normocephalic, no lumps, no lesions, no tenderness.
Face: Symmetrical, no weakness, no involuntary movements.

Eyes

1. Test visual fields by confrontation (cranial nerve II).
2. Test extraocular muscles (EOMs): corneal light reflex, six cardinal positions of gaze (cranial nerves III, IV, VI).
3. Inspect external eye structures.
4. Inspect conjunctivae, sclerae, corneae, irides.
5. Test pupils: size, response to light and accommodation.

Darken room.

Eyes: Visual fields intact by confrontation. EOMs intact. Brows and lashes present. No ptosis. Conjunctivae clear. Sclerae white, no lesions. PERRLA.
Fundi: Red reflex present bilaterally. Discs flat with sharp margins. Vessels present in all quadrants without crossing defects. Retinal background has even colour with no hemorrhages or exudates. Macula has even colour.

Continued

Sequence	Sample Recording
6. Using an ophthalmoscope, inspect ocular fundus: red reflex, disc, vessels, and retinal background.	

Ears

1. Inspect the external ear: position and alignment, skin condition, and auditory meatus.
2. Move auricle and push tragus for tenderness.
3. With an otoscope, inspect the canal and then the tympanic membrane for colour, position, landmarks, and integrity.
4. Assess hearing with the whispered voice test.

Ears: No masses, lesions, tenderness, or discharge. Both TMs pearly grey with light reflex and landmarks intact, no perforations. Whispered words heard bilaterally.

Nose

1. Inspect the external nose: symmetry, lesions.
2. Inspect facial symmetry (cranial nerve VII).
3. Test the patency of each nostril.
4. With a speculum, inspect the nares: nasal mucosa, septum, and turbinates.

Nose: No deformity. Nares patent. Mucosa pink; no septal deviation or perforation.

Mouth and Throat

1. With a penlight, inspect the mouth: buccal mucosa, teeth and gums, tongue, floor of mouth, palate, and uvula.
2. Grade tonsils, if present.
3. Note mobility of uvula as the patient phonates "ahh," and test gag reflex (cranial nerves IX, X).
4. Ask the patient to stick out the tongue (cranial nerve XII).
5. With a gloved hand, bimanually palpate the mouth (if indicated).

Mouth: Can clench teeth. Mucosa and gingivae pink, no masses or lesions. Teeth in good repair. Tongue protrudes in midline; no tremor.
Throat: Mucosa pink, no lesions. Uvula arises in midline on phonation. Tonsils out. Gag reflex present.

Sequence	Sample Recording

Neck

1. Inspect the neck: symmetry, lumps, and pulsations.
2. Palpate the cervical lymph nodes.
3. Inspect and palpate the carotid pulse, one side at a time. Listen for carotid bruits (if indicated).
4. Palpate the trachea in midline.
5. Test ROM and muscle strength against your resistance: head forward and back, head turned to each side, and shoulder shrug (cranial nerve XI).

Neck: Supple with full ROM, no pain. Symmetrical, no lymphade-nopathy or masses; trachea midline; thyroid not palpable, no bruits. Carotid pulses 2 + and = bilaterally.

Step behind the patient, taking your stethoscope, ruler, and marking pen with you.

6. Palpate thyroid gland, posterior approach.

Open the patient's gown to expose all of the back, but leave gown on shoulders and anterior chest.

Chest, Posterior and Lateral

Note: When auscultating breath sounds, do *not* listen over the patient's gown.

1. Inspect the posterior chest: configuration of the thoracic cage, skin characteristics, and symmetry of shoulders and muscles.
2. Palpate for symmetrical expansion, tactile fremitus, lumps, or tenderness.
3. Palpate length of spinous processes.
4. Percuss over all lung fields, noting diaphragmatic excursion.
5. Percuss costovertebral angle, noting tenderness.
6. Auscultate breath sounds, comparing side with side in upper and lateral lung fields; note adventitious sounds.

Chest: AP < transverse diameter. Respirations 16 per minute, relaxed and even. Chest expansion symmetrical. Tactile fremitus sign bilaterally. Resonant to percussion over lung fields. Diaphragmatic excursion 5 cm and = bilaterally. Breath sounds clear. No adventitious sounds.

Move around to face the patient; the patient remains sitting. For a female breast examination, ask permission to lift the gown to drape on the shoulders, exposing the anterior chest; for a male, lower the gown to the lap.

Continued

Sequence	Sample Recording

Chest, Anterior

1. Inspect respirations and skin characteristics.
2. Palpate for tactile fremitus, lumps, or tenderness.
3. Percuss anterior lung fields.
4. Auscultate breath sounds, comparing side with side in upper and lateral lung fields; note adventitious sounds.

Heart

Note: When auscultating heart sounds, do *not* listen over the patient's gown.

1. Ask the patient to lean forward slightly and exhale briefly; auscultate base of the heart for any murmurs.

(See Sample Recording in HEART section following.)

Upper Extremities

1. Test ROM and muscle strength of hands, arms, and shoulders.
2. Palpate the epitrochlear nodes.
3. Palpate for temperature and capillary refill.
4. Compare radial and brachial pulses.

(See Sample Recording in LOWER EXTREMITIES section following.)

Female Breasts

1. Inspect for symmetry, mobility, and dimpling as the patient lifts arms over the head, puts the hands on the hips, and leans forward.
2. Inspect supraclavicular and infraclavicular areas.

Breasts symmetrical. No retraction, no nipple discharge, no lesions. Contour and consistency firm and homogeneous. No masses or tenderness. No lymphadenopathy.

Help the patient to lie supine with their head flat or up to a 30-degree angle. Stand at the patient's right side. Drape the gown up across the shoulders and place an extra sheet across the lower abdomen.

Sequence	Sample Recording

3. Palpate each breast, lifting the same-side arm up over the head. Include the tail of Spence and areola.
4. Palpate each nipple for discharge.
5. Support the patient's arm and palpate the axilla and regional lymph nodes.
6. Teach breast self-examination, if patient asks to learn it.

Male Breasts

1. Inspect and palpate the chest wall.
2. Supporting each arm, palpate the axilla and regional nodes.

Neck Vessels

1. Inspect each side of neck for a jugular venous pulse, turning the patient's head slightly to the other side.
2. Estimate the jugular venous pressure (if indicated).

External jugular veins flat.

Heart

1. Inspect the precordium for pulsations or heave (lift).
2. Palpate the apical impulse, and note the location.
3. Palpate the precordium for thrills.
4. Auscultate the apical rate and rhythm.
5. Auscultate heart sounds with the diaphragm of the stethoscope, inching from the apex up to the base, or vice versa.
6. Auscultate the heart sounds with the bell of the stethoscope, again inching through all locations.
7. Turn the patient over to the left side, while again auscultating the apex with the bell.

Precordium: Apical impulse at 5th intercostal space, left midclavicular line. No heave or thrill, rate 68 per minute and rhythm regular, S$_1$ and S$_2$ are normal, not diminished or accentuated, no extra sounds, no murmurs.

The patient should be supine, with the bed or table flat; arrange drapes to expose the abdomen from the chest to the pubis.

Continued

Sequence	Sample Recording

Abdomen

1. Inspect: contour, symmetry, skin characteristics, umbilicus, and pulsations.
2. Auscultate bowel sounds.
3. Auscultate for vascular sounds over the aorta and renal arteries.
4. Percuss all quadrants.
5. Percuss height of the liver span in right midclavicular line.
6. Percuss the location of the spleen.
7. Palpate using light palpation in all quadrants, then deep palpation in all quadrants.
8. Palpate for liver, spleen, kidneys, and for aorta pulsation.
9. Test the abdominal reflexes (if indicated).

Abdomen: Flat, symmetrical with no apparent masses. Skin smooth with no striae, scars, or lesions. Bowel sounds present, no bruits. Tympany to percussion in all 4 quadrants. Liver span 8 cm in right midclavicular line; splenic dullness at 10th intercostal space in left midaxillary line. Abdomen soft to palpation, no organomegaly, no masses, no tenderness.

Inguinal Area

1. Palpate each side of the groin for the femoral pulse and the inguinal nodes.

Lift the drape to expose the legs.

Lower Extremities

1. Inspect symmetry, skin characteristics, and hair distribution.
2. Palpate pulses: popliteal, posterior tibial, and dorsalis pedis.
3. Use Doppler technique to locate peripheral pulses (if indicated).
4. Palpate for temperature and pretibial edema.
5. Separate toes and inspect.
6. Test ROM and muscle strength of hips, knees, ankles, and feet.

Extremities have brown colour with no redness, cyanosis, or any skin lesions. Extremity size symmetrical with no swelling or atrophy. Temperature warm and = bilaterally.
All pulses present, 2+ and = bilaterally. No lymphadenopathy.
(See Sample Recording in MUSCULO-SKELETAL section following LOWER EXTREMETIES section.)

Ask the patient to sit up and dangle the legs off the bed or table. Keep the gown on and drape it over the lap.

Sequence	Sample Recording

Musculo-Skeletal

1. Note muscle strength as patient sits up.

Neurological

Note: Testing of cranial nerves II to XII was integrated during head and neck regional examinations.

1. Test sensation in selected areas on face, arms, hands, legs, and feet: superficial pain, light touch, and vibration.
2. Test position sense of finger, one hand.
3. Test stereognosis, using a familiar object.
4. Evaluate cerebellar function of the upper extremities with the finger-to-nose test or rapid alternating movements (RAM) test.
5. Elicit deep tendon reflexes of upper extremities: biceps, triceps, and brachioradialis.
6. Test the cerebellar function of the lower extremities by asking the patient to run each heel down the opposite shin.
7. Elicit deep tendon reflexes of the lower extremities: patellar and Achilles.
8. Test the Babinski reflex.

Neurological, sensory: Pinprick, light touch, vibration intact. Stereognosis: Able to identify key.

Motor: No atrophy, weakness, or tremors.

RAM test: Finger-to-nose smoothly intact.

Reflexes: Normal abdominal, DTRs all 2+ and sign bilaterally, no Babinski sign.

Ask the patient to stand with the gown on. Stand close to the patient.

Lower Extremities

1. Inspect lower legs for varicose veins.

Continued

Sequence	Sample Recording

Musculo-Skeletal

1. Ask the patient to walk across the room in his or her regular gait, turn, then walk back toward you in heel-to-toe manner.
2. Ask the patient to walk on the toes for a few steps, then to walk on the heels for a few steps.
3. Stand close, and check for the Romberg sign.
4. Ask the patient to hold the edge of the bed, stand on one leg, and perform a shallow knee bend, one for each leg.
5. Stand behind the patient and check the spine as the patient touches the toes.
6. Stabilize the patient's pelvis and test ROM of the spine as the patient hyperextends, rotates, and laterally bends.

Musculo-skeletal: Gait smooth and fluid, able to tandem walk, no Romberg sign. Joints and muscles symmetrical; no swelling, masses, or deformity; normal spinal curvature. No tenderness to palpation of joints; no heat, swelling, or masses. Full ROM; movement smooth, no crepitance, no tenderness. Muscle strength: Able to maintain flexion against resistance and without tenderness.

Sit on a stool in front of a male patient. The patient stands.

Male Genitalia

1. Inspect the penis and scrotum.
2. Palpate the scrotal contents. If a mass exists, transilluminate the scrotum.
3. Check for inguinal hernia.
4. Teach testicular self-examination.

Male genitalia: No lesions, no inflammation or discharge from penis. Scrotum: Testes descended, symmetrical, no masses. No inguinal hernia.

For an adult male, ask him to bend over the examination table, supporting the torso with his forearms on the table. Assist a bedridden man to a left lateral position with his right leg drawn up. The examiner stands.

Sequence	Sample Recording

Male Rectum

1. Inspect the perianal area.
2. With a gloved, lubricated finger, palpate the rectal walls and prostate gland.
3. Save a stool specimen for an occult blood test.

Rectum: No fissures, hemorrhoids, fistulas, or skin lesions in perianal area. Sphincter tone good, no prolapse. Rectal walls smooth, no masses or tenderness. Prostate not enlarged, no masses or tenderness. Stool brown, guaiac negative.

For an adult female, assist her back to the examination table and help her assume the lithotomy position. Drape her appropriately. Examiner sits on a stool at the foot of the table for the speculum examination, then stands for the bimanual examination.

Female Genitalia

1. Inspect the perineal and perianal areas.
2. Using a vaginal speculum, inspect the cervix and vaginal walls.
3. Procure specimens.
4. Perform a bimanual examination: cervix, uterus, and adnexa.
5. Continue the bimanual examination, checking the rectum and rectovaginal walls.
6. Save a stool specimen for occult blood test.
7. Wipe the perineal area with tissues, and help her up to a sitting position.

External genitalia: No swelling, lesions, or discharge. No urethral swelling or discharge. Internal genitalia: Vaginal walls have no bulging or lesions; cervix pink with no lesions, scant clear mucoid discharge. Bimanual: No pain on moving cervix; uterus anteflexed and anteverted. Adnexa: Ovaries not enlarged.

Rectum: No hemorrhoids, fissures, or lesions; no masses or tenderness. Stool brown, guaiac negative.

Tell the patient you are finished with the examination and that you will leave the room as he or she gets dressed. Return to discuss the examination and further plans and answer any questions. Thank the patient for his or her time.

For the hospitalized patient, return the bed and any room equipment to the way you found it. Make sure the call light and telephone are within easy reach.

Continued

Sequence	Sample Recording

Recording the Data

Record the data from the history and physical examination as soon after the event as possible. Memory fades over time, especially when you are responsible for the care of more than one patient.

It is difficult to strike a balance between recording too much data and recording too little. It is important to remember that from a legal perspective, if a procedure is not documented, it was not performed. Data important for the diagnosis and treatment of the patient's health should be recorded, as well as data that contribute to your decision-making process. This includes charting relevant normal or negative findings.

On the other hand, a listing of every assessment parameter yields an unwieldy, unworkable record. One way to keep your record complete yet succinct is to study your writing style. Use short, clear phrases. Avoid redundant introductory phrases such as, "The patient states that…" Avoid redundant descriptions such as "no inguinal, femoral, or umbilical hernias." Just write "no hernias."

Use simple line drawings to describe your findings. You do not need artistic talent; draw a simple sketch of a tympanic membrane, breast, abdomen, or cervix and mark your findings on it. A clear picture is worth many words.

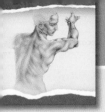
Bedside Assessment and Electronic Health Recording

In a hospital setting, the patient does not require a complete head-to-toe physical examination during every 24-hour stay. The patient *does* require a consistent specialized exam at least every 8 hours that focuses on certain parameters. Note that some measurements, such as daily weights, abdominal girth, or the circumference of a limb, must be measured very carefully. The utility of such measurements depends entirely on consistency from nurse to nurse, for example, use of the same scale for daily weights and same time of day. For patients who do not speak English, obtain a cultural interpreter whenever possible to ensure accuracy of communication.

In addition, remember that many assessments must be performed frequently throughout the course of a hospital shift. This chapter outlines the initial assessment that will allow you to get to know your patient. As you perform this sequence, take note of anything that will need continuous monitoring, such as a blood pressure (BP) or pulse oximetry reading that is not what you expect, or breath sounds that suggest a difficult respiratory effort. If there is no protocol in place for a particular assessment situation, then decide for yourself how often you need to check on the patient's status. It is very easy to be distracted by ringing bells and alarms as the shift progresses, but your own judgement about a patient's needs is just as important as any electronic alert or alarm.

SUBJECTIVE AND OBJECTIVE DATA

Sequence	Selected Photos
Assist the patient into bed. The patient is in bed with the bed at a comfortable level for the examiner.	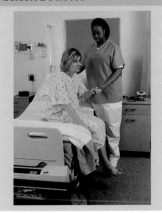

Continued

Sequence	Selected Photos

The Health History

On your way into the patient's room, verify that any necessary markers or flags are in place at the doorway regarding such conditions as isolation precautions, latex allergies, or fall precautions. Once in the room, introduce yourself as the patient's nurse for the next 8 (or 12) hours.

Make direct eye contact and do not allow yourself to be distracted by intravenous (IV) pumps or other equipment as you ask how he or she is feeling, and how he or she spent the previous shift.

Assess for pain: "Are you currently having any pain or discomfort?" You should know when pain medication was most recently administered and what physician orders are written. Determine if further dosing is needed or if you need to contact the physician. With regard to written orders, confirm settings on the patient-controlled analgesia (PCA) pump or epidural setting if one of these is in place. Confirm that the IV solution hanging matches orders for rate and type.

Wash your hands in the patient's presence. Offer water as a courtesy if the patient is allowed water, but also note the physical data this gives you: the patient's ability to hear, follow directions, cross the midline, and ability to swallow. Complete your initial overview by verifying that the correct name band has been applied to the patient's wrist. As you collect this and subsequent history, note data on the general appearance listed below.

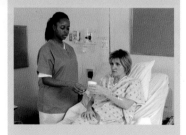

| Sequence | Selected Photos |

General Appearance

1. Facial expression: appropriate for the situation.
2. Body position: relaxed and comfortable or tense and in pain.
3. Level of consciousness: alert and oriented, attentive to your questions, and responding appropriately.
4. Skin colour: even tone consistent with ethnocultural heritage.
5. Nutritional status: weight appears in healthy range, fat distribution is even, hydration appears healthy.
6. Speech: articulation clear and understandable, pattern fluent and even, content appropriate.
7. Hearing: responses and facial expression consistent with what you have said.
8. Personal hygiene: ability to attend to hair, makeup, shaving.

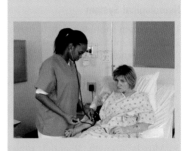

Measurement

1. Measure baseline vital signs (VS): temperature, pulse, respirations, BP. Note which arm to avoid for BP because of surgery, mastectomy, IV access, or dialysis shunt. Collect and document VS more frequently if patient is unstable or if patient condition changes.
2. Measure oxygen saturation (pulse oximetry): maintain at ≥92%, or as ordered (e.g., 88% to 92% for patients with chronic obstructive pulmonary disease [COPD]).
3. Ask the patient to rate pain level on a scale of 0 to 10, at rest and with activity. Note location and quality of pain.
4. Assess pain intensity on scale of 0 to 10 before and after administration of analgesics. Note response according to known pharmacokinetics of the analgesic, approximately 15 minutes after IV administration and 1 hour after oral administration.

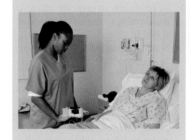

Continued

Sequence	Selected Photos

Neurological System

1. Eyes open spontaneously to name.
2. Verbal responses make sense; speech is clear and articulate.
3. Right (R) and left (L) pupil sizes in millimetres; assess reaction to light.
4. Motor response in upper and lower extremities strong and equal bilaterally.
5. Muscle strength, R and L upper extremities, using hand grips.
6. Muscle strength, R and L lower extremities, pushing feet against your palms.
7. Any ptosis or facial droop.
8. Sensation (omit unless indicated).
9. Ability to swallow.

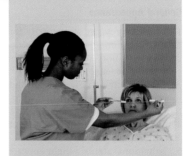

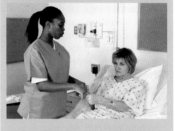

Respiratory System

1. If receiving oxygen by mask or nasal prongs, check fitting and assess skin integrity.
2. Note fraction of inspired oxygen (FiO_2).
3. Respiratory effort.
4. Inquire whether short of breath at rest or on exertion.
5. Auscultate breath sounds, comparing side to side:
   Anterior lobes: right upper, left upper, right middle and lower, left lower
   Posterior lobes: left upper, right upper, left lower, right lower (Note: if not able to sit up, have another nurse hold patient side to side.)
6. Cough and deep breathe; any mucus? Check colour and amount.
7. Incentive spirometer if ordered: encourage patient to use every hour for 10 inspirations. If oxygen saturation or respiratory rate drops, encourage use every 15 minutes.

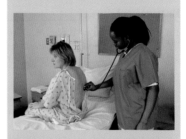

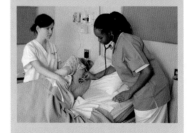

Sequence	Selected Photos

Cardiovascular System

1. Auscultate rhythm at apex: regular, irregular? (Do *not* listen over patient's gown.)
2. Check apical pulse against radial pulse, noting perfusion of all beats.
3. Assess heart sounds in all auscultatory areas: first with diaphragm, repeat with bell.
4. Check capillary refill for prompt return.
5. Check pretibial edema.
6. Palpate the posterior tibial and dorsalis pedis pulses in both feet. (Assess pulses in the lower extremities by Doppler technique, if not palpable.)
7. Verify that the correct IV solution is hanging and flowing at the correct rate according to physician's orders, your own assessment of patient needs.

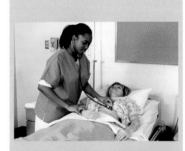

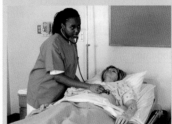

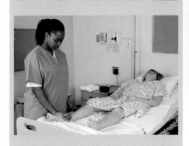

Skin

1. Note skin colour and its consistency with patient's ethnocultural heritage.
2. Palpate skin temperature; expect warm and dry.
3. Pinch a fold of skin under the clavicle or on the forearm to note mobility and turgor.
4. Note skin integrity, any lesions, and the condition of any dressings. Note any bleeding or infection, but do not change dressing until after physical exam.

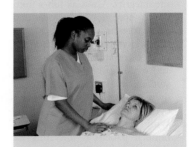

Continued

Sequence	Selected Photos
5. Note date on IV site and note surrounding skin condition (redness, edema, drainage, etc.).	

6. Complete any standardized scales used to quantify the risk of skin breakdown (see Braden Scale for Predicting Pressure Sore Risk, Table 13.1, page 230, in Jarvis: *Physical Examination & Health Assessment*, 3rd Canadian edition).

7. Verify that any air loss or alternating pressure mattress being used are properly applied and operating at the correct settings.

Abdomen

1. Assess contour of abdomen: flat, rounded, protuberant.
2. Listen to bowel sounds in all four quadrants.
3. Perform light palpation in all four quadrants.
4. Inquire whether nauseated or vomiting.
5. Inquire whether the patient is passing flatus or stool, or experiencing constipation or diarrhea. Note date of most recent bowel movement.
6. Check any drainage tube placement for colour, consistency, odour, amount of drainage, and insertion site integrity. Assess all tubes from site to source for kinks, leaks, and disconnections.
7. Check any stoma for colour, moisture, excoriation, and bleeding, and evaluate the integrity of the stomal appliance. Check stomal drainage for colour, consistency, odour, and amount.
8. With regard to diet orders, determine if patient is tolerating ice chips, liquids, solids. Order correct diet as it is advanced. Note if patient is high risk for nutrition deficit.

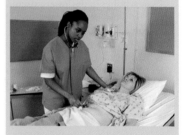

Sequence	Selected Photos

Genitourinary System

1. Inquire whether voiding regularly. Assess indwelling urinary catheter, if indicated.
2. Check urine for colour, clarity.
3. If catheter is in place, check urine colour, quantity, clarity with every VS check.
4. If urine output is below the expected value, perform a bladder scan according to agency protocol. Is the problem in the production of urine or its retention?

Activity

1. With regard to activity orders, if on bed rest, head of bed should be ≥15 degrees. Is patient at high risk for skin breakdown?
2. If ambulatory, assist patient to sitting position, move to chair if no orthostatic hypotension and dizziness; increase activity as tolerated.
3. Note any assistance needed, how tolerates movement, distance walked to chair, ability to turn, steadiness and symmetry of gait.
4. Note any need for any ambulatory aid or equipment.
5. Complete any standardized scales used to quantify the patient's risk for falling and/or functional status, need for referral to physiotherapy or occupational therapy.
6. If anti-embolism compression (TED) stockings and sequential compression devices (SCDs) are ordered, must be on patient 22 hours out of 24 hours to be effective. SCDs must be hooked up and turned on, except during ambulation.

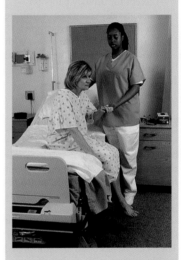

Continued

Sequence	Selected Photos

Report Critical Findings

Note exam findings requiring immediate attention:

1. Altered level of consciousness, confusion
2. Systolic BP ≤90 or ≥160 mm Hg
3. Temperature ≥38°C
4. Heart rate ≤60 or ≥100 bpm
5. Respiratory rate ≤10 per minute or ≥28 per minute
6. Oxygen saturation ≤92%
7. Urine output <30 mL/h for 2 hours
8. Dark amber urine or bloody urine (except for urology patients)
9. Postoperative nausea or vomiting not relieved with medication
10. Surgical pain not controlled with medication; any other unusual pain, such as chest pain
11. Bleeding
12. Sudden restlessness or anxiety

Electronic Health Recording

Most hospitals or clinics now use a basic or a comprehensive **electronic charting system** to replace paper medical records. **Electronic health records (EHRs)** are secure and private lifetime records that describe a person's health history and care (Office of the Auditor General of Canada, 2010). They can be accessed by authorized health professionals and staff across more than one health care organization. Nurses use EHRs in day-to-day practice to review orders, diagnostic test results, dictated notes and consults, and to document nursing care provided, including administration of medications (Furlong, 2015). The structure imposed by the computerized database can serve as a prompt to guide nurses through a complete assessment, and documentation time can be decreased through the use of check boxes and drop-down menus.

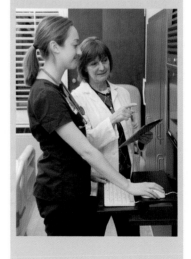

Sequence	Selected Photos
An **electronic medical record (EMR)** is an electronic record of health information that is specific to a single health care organization or clinician's practice, and is often integrated with scheduling and billing software (Canadian Association of Schools of Nursing, 2015). Benefits of EHRs and EMRs include improved legibility and ability to find, search, and share client records. The meaningful use of EHRs and EMRs, which include physician order entry and clinical decision support, may increase patient safety and quality care.	

USING THE SBAR TECHNIQUE FOR STAFF COMMUNICATION

Throughout this text we have used the SOAP acronym (*subjective*, *objective*, *assessment*, *plan*) to organize assessment findings into written or charted communication. To organize assessment data for *verbal* communication (e.g., calls to physicians, nursing shift reports, patient transfers to other units), we use the SBAR framework: *situation*, *background*, *assessment*, *recommendation*.

The SBAR is a structured communication technique to standardize communication and prevent misunderstandings. Communication errors contribute to most patient safety incidents and medical errors in health care (Leonard, Graham, & Bonacum, 2004). Thus, SBAR is used at health care facilities all over the country to improve verbal communication and reduce medical errors (Canadian Patient Safety Institute, 2011; Thomas, Bertram, & Johnson, 2009; Trentham et al., 2010). SBAR is a standardized framework to transmit important, in-the-moment information. Using SBAR will keep your message concise and focused on the immediate problem, yet give your colleagues enough information to understand the current situation and make a decision. To formulate your verbal message, use these four points:

Situation. What is happening right now? What are you calling about? State your name, your unit, patient's name, room number, patient's problem, when it happened or when it started, how severe it is.

Background. Don't recite the patient's full history since admission. Do state the data pertinent to this moment's problem: admitting diagnosis, relevant co-morbidities, time of admission, code status, and appropriate immediate assessment data (e.g., vital signs, pulse oximetry, change in mental status, allergies, current medications, IV fluids, lab results).

Assessment. What do *you* think is happening in regard to the current problem? If you do not know, at least state which body system you think is involved. How severe is the problem?

Recommendation. What do you want the physician to do to improve the patient's situation? Offer probable solutions. Order more pain medication? Come and assess the patient?

Review the following examples of SBAR communication.

Situation 1

S: This is Bill on the Oncology Unit. I'm calling about Daniel Meyers in room 8417. He is refusing all oral medications as of now.

B: Daniel is a 59-year-old male with multiple myeloma. He was admitted for an autologous stem cell transplant and received chemotherapy 10 days ago. Now he is 5 days post-transplantation. Vital signs are stable, alert, and oriented, IVs are D$_5$W [5% dextrose in water]. As of 1 hour ago, he has been feeling extreme nausea and vomiting, refusing all food and oral meds.

A: I think the chemo he had pre-transplant is hitting him now. His uncontrolled nausea isn't going away in the next few days.

R: I'm concerned he cannot stay hydrated, and he needs his meds. I need you to please change the IV rate and change all scheduled oral meds to IV. I also think we need to add an additional PRN (as needed) antiemetic. If he continues to refuse food, we may have to consider starting him on TPN (total parenteral nutrition)/lipids.

Situation 2

S: This is Andrea. I'm the nurse taking care of Max Goodson in 6443. His condition has changed, and his most recent vital signs show a significant drop in BP.

B: Max is 40 years old with a history of alcoholism. He was admitted through the ED last night with abdominal pain and suspected GI (gastro-intestinal) bleeding. His BPs have been running in the 130s/80s. He just produced a large amount of liquid maroon stool and reported feeling dizzy. I rechecked his vitals, and his BP is 88/50 and heart rate is 104.

A: I'm worried his GI bleed is getting worse.

R: Will you order a stat CBC (complete blood cell count) and place an order to transfuse RBCs (red blood cells) if his Hgb (hemoglobin) is below 8 mg? Also, can you please come and assess? I think we may need to insert an NG (nasogastric) tube and do lavage.

ILLUSTRATION CREDITS

Chapter 1

Figure 1.1: Adapted from the American Society of Human Genetics (2004). Retrieved from www.ashg.org.

Chapter 2

Figure 2.1: Retrieved from http://www.mocatest.org/pdf_files/test/MoCA-Test-English_7_1.pdf. Copyright © Dr. Z. Nasreddine, 2003 to 2012: *The Montreal Cognitive Assessment* (MoCA). All rights reserved. Reprinted with permission.

Chapter 4

Figure 4.1: Health Canada. (2003). *Canadian guidelines for body weight classifications in adults* (Catalogue No. H49-179/2003E; p. 37). Ottawa: Author. Retrieved from http://www.hc-sc.gc.ca/fn-an/alt_formats/hpfb-dgpsa/pdf/nutrition/weight_book-livres_des_poids_e.pdf.

Figure 4.4: Canadian Hypertension Education Program (CHEP). (2017). Hypertension Canada's 2017 Guidelines for Diagnosis, Risk Assessment, Prevention, and Treatment of Hypertension in Adults. *Canadian Journal of Cardiology*, 33(5), 557–576.

Chapter 5

Figure 5.1: Lewis, S. L., Dirksen, S. R., Heitkemper, et al. (2011). *Medical-surgical nursing: Assessment and management of clinical problems* (8th ed., p. 437, Figure 23.1). St. Louis: Mosby.

Unnumbered figures in Table 5.3: Copyright Pat Thomas, 2010.

Unnumbered figures in Table 5.4: Copyright Pat Thomas, 2010.

Unnumbered figures in Table 5.5: From Potter, P.A., & Perry, A.G. (2009). *Fundamentals of nursing*

(7th ed., p. 1283, Fig. 48.6). St. Louis, Mosby.

Chapter 7

Figure 7.1: Copyright Pat Thomas, 2006.

Figure 7.3: Courtesy Heather Boyd-Monk and Wills Eye Hospital, Philadelphia, PA.

Unnumbered figures in Table 7.1: Copyright Pat Thomas, 2010.

Unnumbered figures in Table 7.2: Ptosis (Drooping Upper Eyelid); Hordeolum; Conjunctivitis: Courtesy Lemmi & Lemmi, 2011; **Ectropion and Entropion:** From Albert, D. M., & Jakobiec, F. A. (1994). *Principles and practice of ophthalmology* (vol. 3, p. 1849). Philadelphia: Saunders; **Chalazion:** Courtesy Heather Boyd-Monk and Wills Eye Hospital, Philadelphia, PA; **Basal Cell Carcinoma:** From Scheie, H. G., & Albert, D. M. (1977). *Textbook of ophthalmology* (9th ed., p. 449). Philadelphia: Saunders.

Chapter 8

Figure 8.1: Courtesy Lemmi & Lemmi, 2011.

Figure 8.2: Copyright Pat Thomas, 2010.

Unnumbered figures in Table 8.1: Excessive Cerumen and Otitis Externa (Swimmer's Ear): Copyright Pat Thomas, 2010; **Retracted Eardrum:** From Adams, G. L., Boies, L. R., & Hilger, P. A. (1989). *Boies fundamentals of otolaryngology: A textbook of ear, nose, and throat diseases* (6th ed., p. 6). Philadelphia: W. B. Saunders; **Acute (Purulent) Otitis Media:** From Adams, G. L., Boies, L. R., & Hilger, P. A. (1989). *Boies fundamentals of otolaryngology: A textbook of ear, nose, and throat diseases* (6th ed.). Philadelphia: W. B.

Saunders; **Otitis Media with Effusion and Perforation:** From Swartz, M. H. (2010). *Textbook of physical diagnosis: History and examination* (6th ed., p. 320, Fig. 11.34A and p. 318, Fig. 11.30A). Philadelphia: W. B. Saunders.

Chapter 9

Figures 9.1 and 9.2: Copyright Pat Thomas, 2006.

Figure 9.3: Copyright Pat Thomas, 2010.

Unnumbered figures in Table 9.1: Foreign Body; Acute Rhinitis; and Allergic Rhinitis: From Fireman, P. (1996). *Atlas of allergies* (2nd ed.). London: Mosby; **Perforated Septum:** From Hawke, M. (1998). *Diagnostic handbook of otorhinolaryngology.* London: Martin Dunitz (p. 122, Fig. 2.60). Reproduced by permission of Taylor & Francis Books UK.

Unnumbered figures in Table 9.2: Angular Cheilitis (Stomatitis, Perlèche): From Callen, J. P., Greer, K. E., Hood, A. F., et al. (1993). *Color Atlas of Dermatology* (p. 326). Philadelphia: W.B. Saunders; **Gingivitis:** From Callen, J. P., Greer, K. E., Hood, A. F., et al. (1993). *Color Atlas of Dermatology* (p. 385). Philadelphia: W. B. Saunders; **Herpes Simplex I:** Courtesy Lemmi & Lemmi, 2011; **Aphthous Ulcers:** from Sleisinger, M. H., & Fordtran, J. S. (1993). *Gastrointestinal Diseases: Pathophysiology, Diagnosis, and Management* (5th ed., vol. 1, colour plate WVII-B). Philadelphia: Saunders; **Torus Palatinus:** from Ibsen, O A. C., & Phelen, J. A. *Oral Pathology for the Dental Hygienist,* (2nd ed., slide 284). Philadelphia: Saunders; **Acute Tonsillitis and Pharyngitis:** Courtesy Lemmi & Lemmi, 2011.

Chapter 10

Figures 10.1 and 10.2: Copyright Pat Thomas, 2010.

Chapter 11

Figures 11.1 and 11.2: Copyright Pat Thomas, 2010.

Chapter 12

Figures 12.1 and 12.2: Copyright Pat Thomas, 2006.

Unnumbered figures in Table 12.2: Copyright Pat Thomas, 2006.

Chapter 13

Figures 13.1, 13.2, and 13.3: Copyright Pat Thomas, 2010.

Chapter 14

Figures 14.1, 14.2, and 14.5: Copyright Pat Thomas, 2006.

Chapter 15

Figure 15.2: Copyright Pat Thomas, 2006.

Figure 15.9: Courtesy Lemmi & Lemmi, 2011.

Unnumbered figures in Table 15.2: Scoliosis *(top):* Courtesy Lemmi & Lemmi, 2011; **Scoliosis *(bottom):*** Zitelli, B. J., McIntire, S. C., & Nowalk, A. J. (2012). *Zitelli & Davis' atlas of pediatric physical diagnosis* (6th ed., p. 840, Figure 21.71B). St. Louis: Mosby; **Herniated Nucleus Pulposus:** From Polley, H. F., & Hunder, G. G. (1978). *Rheumatologic interviewing and physical examination of the joints* (2nd ed.). Philadelphia: W. B. Saunders.

Chapter 16

Figures 16.1, 16.2, 16.3, and 16.4: Copyright Pat Thomas, 2006.
Figure 16.19: Copyright Pat Thomas, 2014.

Chapter 17

Figure 17.1: Copyright Pat Thomas, 2010.
Unnumbered figures in Table 17.1: Copyright Pat Thomas, 2006.

Chapter 19

Figure 19.1: Copyright Pat Thomas, 2010.

Chapter 21

Unnumbered figures in selected photos From Potter, P. A., Perry, A. G., Stockert, P., Hall, A. (2015). *Essentials for Nursing Practice* (8th ed.). St. Louis: Mosby.

REFERENCES

Arthritis Society. (2015). *Types of arthritis*. Retrieved from http://arthritis.ca/understand-arthritis/types-of-arthritis.

Bellaud, G., Canestri, A., Gallah, S., et al. (2017). Bacterial chondritis complications following ear piercing. *Médecine et maladies infectieuses, 47*(1), 26–31. Retrieved from http://dx.doi.org/10.1016/j.medmal.2016.07.002.

Blacquiere, D., Lindsay, P., Foley, N., et al. (2017). Canadian stroke best practice recommendations: Telestroke best practice guidelines update 2017. *Inter J Stroke, 12*(8), 886–895. doi:10.1177/1747493017706239.

Bournes, A. (2015). *Guidelines and protocols for hormone therapy and primary health care for trans clients*. Retrieved from http://sherbourne.on.ca/lgbt-health/guidelines-protocols-for-trans-care/.

Canadian Academy of Health Sciences. (2014). *Improving access to oral health care for vulnerable people living in Canada*. Retrieved from http://cahs-acss.ca/wp-content/uploads/2015/07/Access_to_Oral_Care_FINAL_REPORT_EN.pdf.

Canadian Association of Schools of Nursing. (2015). *Nursing informatics: Entry-to-practice competencies for registered nurses*. Ottawa: Author. Retrieved from https://www.casn.ca/wp-content/uploads/2014/12/Nursing-Informatics-Entry-to-Practice-Competencies-for-RNs_updated-June-4-2015.pdf.

Canadian Cancer Society. (2017). *Lung cancer statistics*. Retrieved from http://www.cancer.ca/en/cancer-information/cancer-type/lung/statistics/?region=on.

Canadian Cancer Society. (2017a). *Screening for breast cancer*. Retrieved from http://www.cancer.ca/en/cancer-information/cancer-type/breast/screening/?region=bc.

Canadian Cancer Society. (2017b). *Testicular cancer*. Retrieved from http://www.cancer.ca/en/cancer-information/cancer-type/testicular/testicular-cancer/?region=on.

Canadian Cancer Statistics Advisory Committee. (2017). *Canadian Cancer Statistics 2017*. Toronto, ON: Canadian Cancer Society. Available at: cancer.ca/Canadian-Cancer-Statistics-2018-EN. (Accessed 7 July 2018).

Canadian Hypertension Education Program (CHEP). (2016). Guidelines for Blood Pressure Measurement, Diagnosis, Assessment of Risk, Prevention, and Treatment of Hypertension. *Canadian Journal of Cardiology, 32*(5), 569–588.

Canadian Ophthalmological Society Clinical Practice Guideline Expert Committee (COSCPGEC). (2007). Canadian Ophthalmological Society evidence-based clinical practice guidelines for the periodic eye examination in adults in Canada. *Canadian Journal of Ophthalmology, 42*, 39–45.

Canadian Patient Safety Institute (2011). *Canadian framework for teamwork and communication: Literature review, needs assessment, evaluation of training tools and expert consultations*. Edmonton: Author. Retrieved from http://www.patientsafetyinstitute.ca/en/toolsResources/teamworkCommunication/Documents/Canadian%20Framework%20for%20Teamwork%20and%20Communications.pdf.

Canadian Paediatric Society (2014). *Promoting optimal monitoring of child growth in Canada: Using the new who growth charts*. Retrieved from http://www.cps.ca/uploads/tools/growth-charts-statement-FULL.pdf.

Denny, K., Lawand, C., & Perry, S. (2013). Compromised wounds in

Canada. *Healthcare Quarterly, 17*(1), 7–10. doi:10.12927/hcq.2014.23787.

Duval Smith, F. (2016). Caring for surgical patients with piercings. *Association of periOperative Nurses Journal, 103*(6), 584–593. doi:10.1016/j.aorn.2016.04.005.

Epp, A., & Larochelle, A. (2010). SOGC clinical practice guideline: Recurrent urinary tract infection. *Journal of Obstetrics and Gynaecology Canada, 250*, 1082–1090.

Fischer, M., Rüegg, S., Czaplinski, A., et al. (2010). Inter-rater reliability of the Full Outline of UnResponsiveness score and the Glasgow Coma Scale in critically ill patients: A prospective observational study. *Critical Care* (London, England), *14*(2), R64. Retrieved from http://ccforum.com/content/14/2/R64.

Furlong, K. E. (2015). Learning to use an EHR: Nurses' stories. *Canadian Nurse, 111*(5), 20–24.

Gallant, V., Duccuri, V., & McGuire, M. (2017). Tuberculosis in Canada—summary 2015. *Canada Communicable Disease Report, 43*(3), 77–82. Retrieved from https://www.canada.ca/content/dam/phac-aspc/migration/phac-aspc/publicat/ccdr-rmtc/17vol43/dr-rm43-3-4/assets/pdf/17vol43_3_4-ar-04-eng.pdf.

Government of Canada. (2017). *Heart disease in Canada: Highlights from the Canadian Chronic Disease Surveillance System.* Retrieved from https://www.canada.ca/en/public-health/services/publications/diseases-conditions/heart-disease-canada-fact-sheet.html.

Government of Canada. (2018). *Surveillance of heart diseases and conditions.* Retrieved from https://www.canada.ca/en/public-health/services/diseases/heart-health/heart-diseases-conditions/surveillance-heart-diseases-conditions.html.

Health Canada. (2016). *Canadian guidelines for body weight classifications in adults—quick reference tools for professionals.* Retrieved from http://www.hc-sc.gc.ca/fn-an/nutrition/weights-poids/guide-ld-adult/cg_quick_ref-ldc_rapide_ref-eng.php.

Holzhauer, J. K., Reith, V., Sawin, K. J., et al. (2009). Evaluation of temporal artery thermometry in children 3–36 months old. *Journal for Specialists in Pediatric Nursing, 14*(4), 239–244.

Jayasinghe, Y., & Simmons, P. S. (2009). Fibroadenomas in adolescence. *Current Opinion in Obstetrics & Gynecology, 21*(5), 402–406. doi:10.1097/GCO.0b013e32832fa06b.

Jin, Y.-P., & Trope, G. E. (2011). Eye care utilization in Canada: Disparity in the publicly funded health care system. *Canadian Journal of Ophthalmology/Journal Canadien d'Ophtalmologie, 46*(2), 133–138. doi:10.3129/i10-120.

Leonard, M., Graham, S., & Bonacum, D. (2004). The human factor: The critical importance of effective teamwork and communication in providing safe care. *Quality and Safety in Health Care, 13*(Suppl. 1), i85–i90.

Lin, S. N., Taylor, J., Alperstein, S., et al. (2014). Does speculum lubricant affect liquid-based Papanicolaou test adequacy? *Cancer Cytopathology, 122*, 221–226. doi:10.1002/cncy.21369.

Love, S., & Lindsey, K. (2015). *Dr. Susan Love's breast book* (6th ed.). Cambridge, MA: Da Capo Lifelong Books.

McCaffery, M. (1968). *Nursing practice theories related to cognition, bodily pain, and man-environment interactions.* Los Angeles: University of California.

McGee, S. (2018). *Evidence-based physical diagnosis* (4th ed.). Philadelphia: Saunders.

National Pressure Ulcer Advisory Panel (NPUAP). (2007). *Pressure ulcer stages revised by NPUAP.* Retrieved September 20, 2009, from www.npuap.org/pr2.htm.

Office of the Auditor General of Canada. (2010). *Electronic health records in Canada: An overview of federal and provincial audit reports.* Retrieved from http://www.oag-bvg.gc.ca/internet/English/parl_oag_201004_07_e_33720.html.

Ontario Stroke Network. (2016). *Stroke stats & facts.* Retrieved from http://ontariostrokenetwork.ca/information-about-stroke/stroke-stats-and-facts/.

Public Health Agency of Canada. (2011). *Chapter 1: Life with arthritis in Canada: A personal and public health challenge—What is arthritis and how common is it?* Retrieved from https://www.canada.ca/en/public-health/services/chronic-diseases/arthritis/life-arthritis-canada-a-personal-public-health-challenge/chapter-one-what-is-arthritis-and-how-common-is-it.html.

Public Health Agency of Canada. (2012). *Routine practices and additional precautions for preventing the transmission of infection in health-care settings.* Retrieved from http://publications.gc.ca/collections//collection_2013/aspc-phac/HP40-83-2013-eng.pdf.

Public Health Agency of Canada. (2015). *Canadian guidelines on sexually transmitted infections: Primary care and sexually transmitted infections.* Retrieved from http://www.phac-aspc.gc.ca/std-mts/sti-its/cgsti-ldcits/section-2-eng.php#a2.

Public Health Agency of Canada (2016). *Health status of Canadians 2016.* Ottawa: Her Majesty the Queen in Right of Canada as represented by the Minister of Health. Retrieved from http://healthycanadians.gc.ca/publications/department-ministere/state-public-health-status-2016-etat-sante-publique-statut/alt/pdf-eng.pdf.

Statistics Canada. (2017). *Health fact sheet: Chronic conditions.* Ottawa: Minister of Industry. Retrieved from http://www.statcan.gc.ca/pub/82-625-x/2017001/article/54858-eng.pdf.

Statistics Canada. (2018). *Leading causes of death, by sex.* Retrieved from http://www.statcan.gc.ca/tables-tableaux/sum-som/l01/cst01/hlth36a-eng.htm.

Storey, J., Rowland, J., Basic, C., et al. (2004). The Rowland Universal Dementia Assessment Scale (RU-DAS): A multicultural cognitive assessment scale. *International Psychogeriatrics, 16*(1), 13–31. Retrieved from https://www.fightdementia.org.au/sites/default/files/20110311_2011RUDASAdminScoringGuide.pdf.

Tarlo, S. M., & Lemiere, C. (2014). Occupational asthma. *New England Journal of Medicine, 370*(7), 640–649.

Thomas, C. M., Bertram, E., & Johnson, D. (2009). The SBAR communication technique. *Nurse Educator, 34*(4), 176–180.

Trentham, B., Andreoli, A., Boaro, N., et al. (2010). *SBAR: A shared structure for effective team communication: An implementation toolkit* (2nd ed.). Toronto: Toronto Rehabilitation Institute.

Tsoi, K. K., Chan, J. Y., Hirai, H. W., et al. (2015). Cognitive test to detect dementia: A systematic review and meta-analysis. *JAMA Internal Medicine, 175*(9), 1450–1458. doi: 10.1001/jamainternmed.2015.2152. Retrieved from https://www.ncbi.nlm.nih.gov/pubmed/26052687.

Walling, A., & Dickson, G. (2012). Hearing loss in older adults.

American Family Physician, 85(12), 1150–1156.

Widschwendter, P., Friedl, T. W., Schwentner, L., et al. (2015). The influence of obesity on survival in early, high-risk breast cancer: Results from the randomized SUCCESS A trial. *Breast Cancer Research, 17,* 129. doi:10.1186/s13058-015-0639-3.

World Health Organization (WHO). (2017). *BMI classification.* Retrieved from http://www.who.int/bmi/index.jsp?introPage=intro_3.html.

INDEX